Recent Results in Cancer Research 116

Recent Results in Cancer Research

Volume 106
E. Grundmann, L. Beck (Eds.): Minimal Neoplasia
1988. 128 figures, 61 tables. IX, 194. ISBN 3-540-18455-4

Volume 107
R. D. Issels, W. Wilmanns (Eds.):
Application of Hyperthermia in the Treatment of Cancer
1988. 118 figures, 56 tables. XII, 277. ISBN 3-540-18486-4

Volume 108
H.-J. Senn, A. Glaus, L. Schmid (Eds.):
Supportive Care in Cancer Patients
1988. 62 figures, 97 tables. XII, 342. ISBN 3-540-17150-9

Volume 109
W. Hinkelbein, G. Bruggmoser, R. Engelhardt (Eds.):
Preclinical Hyperthermia
1988. 182 figures, 40 tables. XI, 261. ISBN 3-540-18487-2

Volume 110
P. Schlag, P. Hohenberger, U. Metzger (Eds.):
Combined Modality Therapy of Gastrointestinal Tract Cancer
1988. 105 figures, 122 tables. XVII, 301. ISBN 3-540-18610-7

Volume 111
H. Scheurlen, R. Kay, M. Baum (Eds.):
Cancer Clinical Trials: A Critical Appraisal
1988. 37 figures, 53 tables. XI, 272. ISBN 3-540-19098-8

Volume 112
L. Schmid, H.-J. Senn (Eds.): AIDS-Related Neoplasias
1988. 23 figures, 35 tables. IX, 97. ISBN 3-540-19227-1

Volume 113
U. Eppenberger, A. Goldhirsch (Eds.):
Endocrine Therapy and Growth Regulation of Breast Cancer
1989. 26 figures, 17 tables. IX, 92. ISBN 3-540-50456-7

Volume 114
E. Grundmann (Ed.): Cancer Mapping
1989. 97 figures, 64 tables. ISBN 3-540-50490-7

Volume 115
H.-J. Senn, A. Goldhirsch, R. D. Gelber, B. Osterwalder (Eds.):
Adjuvant Therapy of Primary Breast Cancer
1989. ISBN 3-540-18810-X

K. W. Brunner H. Fleisch H.-J. Senn (Eds.)

Bisphosphonates and Tumor Osteolysis

With 22 Figures and 6 Tables

Springer-Verlag
Berlin Heidelberg New York
London Paris Tokyo

Professor Dr. Kurt W. Brunner
Institut für Medizinische Onkologie
Inselspital Bern
3010 Bern, Switzerland

Professor Dr. Herbert Fleisch
Pathophysiologisches Institut
Universität Bern
Murtenstraße 35, 3010 Bern, Switzerland

Professor Dr. Hans-Jörg Senn
Medizinische Klinik C
Kantonsspital St. Gallen
9007 St. Gallen, Switzerland

ISBN 3-540-50560-1 Springer-Verlag Berlin Heidelberg New York
ISBN 0-387-50560-1 Springer-Verlag New York Berlin Heidelberg

Typsetting, printing, and binding: Appl, Wemding
2125/3140-543210 - Printed on acid-free paper.

Preface

Skeletal involvement is a frequent and troublesome complication affecting many patients with neoplastic disease, especially multiple myeloma and cancer of the breast, lung, and prostate. This involvement can finally lead to local bone destruction with resulting fractures, local bone neoformation, or hypercalcemia. The latter complicates the clinical course of 10%–20% of the patients with non-small-cell lung cancer and mammary tumors. Both knowledge of the pathophysiologic mechanisms and treatment of this skeletal involvement have progressed substantially in the last years. One of the very recent therapeutic advances has been the finding that bisphosphonates, a family of compounds characterized by a P–C–P bond, are effective in alleviating some of these conditions.

This volume represents the proceedings of a workshop held on December 4, 1987, in Lucerne, Switzerland, devoted to the use of bisphosphonates in tumoral bone disease. This educational workshop was organized by the Swiss Group for Clinical Cancer Research (SAKK) to foster international scientific exchange and to clarify experimental and clinical problems in the therapeutic application of bisphosphonates. Experts from various countries were invited to present and discuss their experimental findings and their preliminary clinical results. This volume summarizes the invited contributions, which will be of major interest to clinical oncologists, surgeons, internists, endocrinologists, and pathologists confronted with bone destruction in neoplastic disease. We acknowledge gratefully the support of Boehringer Mannheim (Schweiz) AG, Rotkreuz.

The first report on the effect of bisphosphonates on bone dates back to 20 years ago (Fleisch et al. 1968),[1] when it was shown that these compounds are powerful inhibitors of mineralization and of bone destruction both in vitro and in the experimental animal.

---

[1] Fleisch H, Russell RGG, Bisaz S, Casey PA, Mühlbauer RC (1968) The influence of pyrophosphate analogues (diphosphonates) on the precipitation and dissolution of calcium phosphate in vitro and in vivo. Calc Tiss Res 2 [Suppl]: 10–10A

Dichloromethylenebisphosphonate seemed particularly interesting: Although quite a potent inhibitor of bone resorption, it has relatively little effect on bone calcification. Later work showed that bisphosphonates inhibit both normal bone disintegration and destruction induced by a variety of causes, e.g., parathyroid hormone, immobilization, and tumors. It was also found that changing the side chains on the C atom of the P–C–P backbone drastically altered the activity, and this discovery stimulated chemists to synthesize new structures. A great number of bisphosphonates have now been tested, and the latest compounds are active when given in amounts as low as 1 μg P per kg in the rat. Although no clear-cut structure–effect relation has yet been established, the effect is thought to be due to the inactivation of the osteoclasts, as well as possibly to the inhibition of the recruitment of these cells. The fact that the bisphosphonates are characteristic "bone seekers" with regard to their strong affinity for hydroxyapatite explains why their activity is almost exclusively restricted to bone.

These findings opened up the possibility of using bisphosphonates in clinical practice. Their strong binding to apatite was the rationale for their worldwide use in nuclear medicine as imaging substances bound to technetium 99m. Their inhibitory effect on mineralization is at the basis of their use in heterotopic ossification and as antitartar agents in toothpastes. However, the most common application of bisphosphonates is in diseases featuring progressive bone destruction. Thus, 1-hydroxyethylidene-1,1-bisphosphonate is now used in many countries for the treatment of Paget's disease.

This book reports new findings on the inhibitory effect of some bisphosphonates, especially dichloromethylenebisphosphonate, on neoplastic hypercalcemia and bone destruction due to neoplastic bone disease. Some of the effects, particularly the short-term ones, are well established.

Others, such as a possible beneficial effect on the long-term development of metastatic bone disease, need confirmation by larger randomized studies. Although the mechanism is not an antitumoral one per se, but a shielding of bone, the increase in quality of life through the decrease in pain and the prevention of hypercalcemia has already made bisphosphonates a most useful auxiliary in the battery of drugs used by oncologists in the treatment of patients with acute tumoral bone disease. Further developments in this exciting new area of treatment are expected in the near future.

K. Brunner
H. Fleisch
H. J. Senn

Contents

*List of Contributors**

* The address of the prinipal authors is given on the first page of each contribution.

[1] Page on which contribution begins.

*Bisphosphonates: A New Class of Drugs in Diseases of Bone and Calcium Metabolism**

H. Fleisch

Department of Pathophysiology, University of Berne, Murtenstraße 35, 3010 Berne, Switzerland

Introduction

The bisphosphonates are a new class of drugs which have been developed in the past 2 decades for use in various diseases of bone, tooth, and calcium metabolism. Three are on the market today, while others are under clinical or preclinical investigation. This chapter will cover chemical and experimental aspects as well as clinical applications of these compounds. Literature is essentially limited to one reference, usually the original report. For two recent reviews, weighted somewhat differently and with more extensive references, see Fleisch (1983) and Francis and Martodam (1983).

Chemistry and General Characteristics

Bisphosphonates, previously erroneously called diphosphonates, are compounds characterized by two C-P bonds. If the two bonds are located on the same carbon atom, the compounds are called geminal bisphosphonates. They are therefore analogs of pyrophosphate, which contains an oxygen instead of a carbon atom.

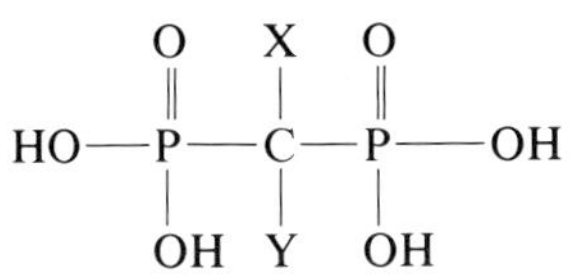

Bisphosphonic acid

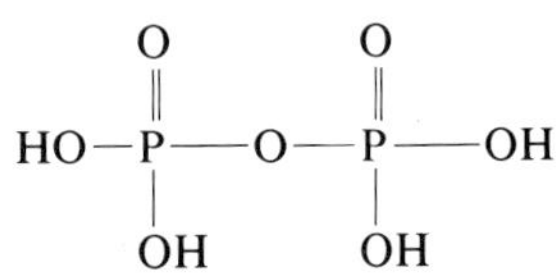

Pyrophosphoric acid

In this chapter, only the geminal bisphosphonates will be discussed, since these have been shown to have the strongest activity in vivo and are the only ones used clinically today, the other types of bisphosphonates being less active or not active at all on bone and calcification. For the sake of simplicity, they will be called just bisphosphonates, although it must be emphasized that this is not entirely correct.

* This chapter has already appeared in *Handbook of Experimental Pharmacology*, vol 83, edited by P. F. Baker, Springer-Verlag Berlin Heidelberg 1988.

Recent Results in Cancer Research, Vol. 116

The basic structure P – C – P allows a great number of possible variations, either by changing the two lateral chains on the carbon atom or by esterifying the phosphate groups. A large number of bisphosphonates can be and have been synthesized. Some of them have been tested biologically. It has emerged that each bisphosphonate has its own physicochemical and biologic characteristics, and this is of great interest in the light of the future development of these compounds. This means, however, that it is not possible to extrapolate from the results of one compound to others without great caution, and that it is not correct to talk generally of the effects of bisphosphonates. It is necessary to consider each bisphosphonate on its own and always to restrict statements to specific compounds.

The P – C – P bond of the bisphosphonates is relatively stable to heat and most chemical reagents and completely resistant to enzymatic hydrolysis. The four dissociation constants vary with the two side chains on the carbon atom, pK_1 being mostly between 1 and 2, pK_2 between 2 and 3, pK_3 between 5 and 8, and pK_4 between 8 and 12 (Curry and Nicholson 1972). The bisphosphonates have a strong affinity for metal ions such as calcium, magnesium, and especially iron (Curry and Nicholson 1972). Some uncertainty still exists as to their state when in solution. Indeed, they are only partially ultrafiltrable in aqueous solutions as well as in plasma (Wiedmer et al. 1983). In the presence of calcium and other metals, the hydroxybisphosphonates can make polynuclear complexes not only at alkaline pH (Grabenstetter and Cilley 1971), but also at physiologic pH (Lamson et al. 1984). Whether this occurs in vivo, and whether this is the cause of the impaired ultrafiltrability, is unknown.

The following bisphosphonates have been investigated in humans, the first three being on the market in certain countries, the former two as an agent against bone disease, the latter for dental use.

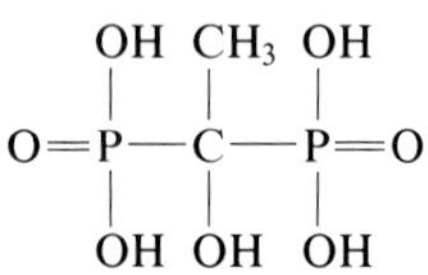

1-Hydroxyethylidene-1,1-bisphosphonic acid (HEBP), previously called ethane-1-hydroxy-1,1-diphosphonic acid (EHDP)

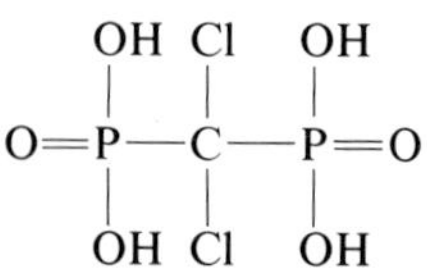

Dichloromethylenebisphosphonic acid (Cl_2MBP), previously called dichloromethylenediphosphonic acid (Cl_2MDP)

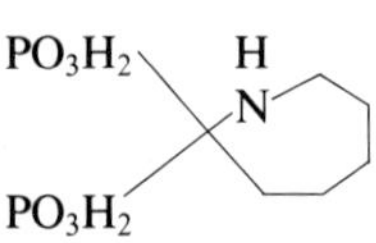

Azacycloheptylidene-2,2-bisphosphonic acid

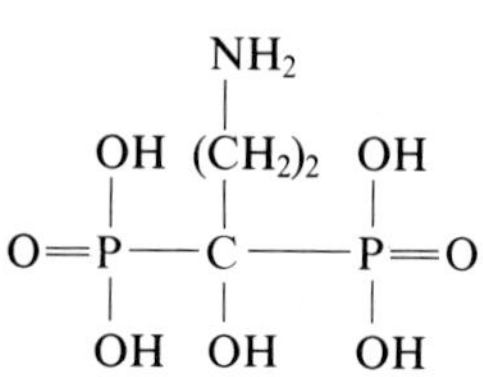

3-Amino-1-hydroxypropylidene-1,1-bisphosphonic acid (AHPrBP), previously called 3-amino-1-hydroxypropane-1,1-diphosphonic acid (APD)

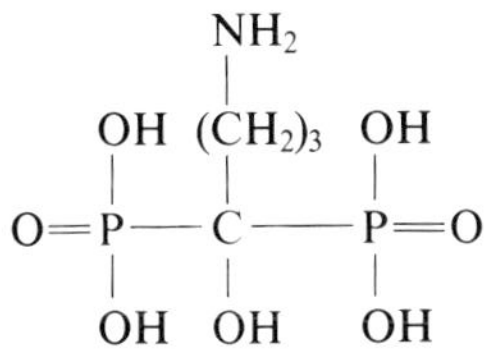

4-Amino-1-hydroxybutylidene-1,1-bisphosphonic acid (AHBuBP)

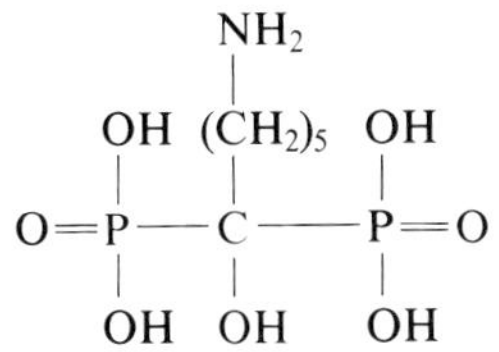

6-Amino-1-hydroxyhexylidene-1,1-bisphosphonic acid (AHHexBP)

Synthesis

The bisphosphonates can be synthesized in a variety of ways (Curry and Nicholson 1972; Worms and Schmidt-Dunker 1976). The commonest method of obtaining 1-hydroxy-1,1-bisphosphonates is the reaction of the corresponding carboxylic acid with a mixture of H_3PO_4 and PCl_3. The products obtained under these anhydrous conditions are condensates, i.e., two or more molecules of the bisphosphonate condensed via the removal of a molecule of water. These condensates can then be converted by heating in water or in 6 *M* HCl. This technique is one of the simplest ways of producing the bisphosphonates HEBP or AHPrBP (Blaser et al. 1971). Another method consists in using a Michaelis-Arbuzov-like reaction (Harvey and De Sombre 1964), whereby a carboxylic acid chloride is made to react with a trialkylphosphite. The resultant acylphosphonate reacts under slightly basic conditions with a dialkylphosphite to yield a bisphosphonate tetraalkyl ester, which can then be hydrolyzed with HCl to the corresponding free acid. The 1-amino-1,1-bisphosphonates are made by reacting a nitrile or an amide with H_3PO_4 and a phosphorus trihalide and hydrolyzing the product with water. The reaction can also be carried out directly in the presence of water (Worms and Blum 1979).

Methods of Determination

Various methods are available to determine the structure and the purity of bisphosphonates and are used in the synthesis of these compounds. They include, among others, nuclear magnetic resonance techniques (H-NMR, ^{13}C-NMR, and P-NMR) and gel electrophoresis. The measurement in biologic fluids or in tissues is, however, more difficult and far from satisfactory. The difficulty arises from the small concentrations present and from the large amounts of inorganic phosphate and various organic phosphates found in biologic samples. For this reason, pharmacodynamics have been performed almost exclusively with radioactively labeled compounds and pharmacokinetic data with unlabeled compounds are very scanty in humans.

One technique (Bisaz et al. 1975a), which permits measurement of HEBP down to 1 nmol, is based on a partial purification of HEBP from organic and inorganic phosphate and measurement of inorganic phosphate production under UV exposure. Another (Liggett 1973) which is, however, much less sensitive, involves titration with thorium diaminocyclohexanetetraacetate in the presence of xylanol orange after purification by means of precipitation on calcium phosphate or calcium hydroxide. Finally, a technique developed for Cl_2MBP (Chester et al. 1981) and which allows the measurement of about 7 nmol is based on flame photometry detection after purification by adsorption onto calcium phosphate and ion exchange chromatography.

Monophosphonates

Since the bisphosphonates are chemically two monophosphonates, a few comments on these latter compounds are relevant. Whereas until now no bisphosphonates have been found to occur naturally in animals or humans, monophosphonates, that is, compounds which have one P–C bond, occur throughout the animal world (Hilderbrand and Henderson 1983). The first, and probably the most important, was detected only in 1959 and identified as 2-aminoethylphosphonic acid (AEP) (Horiguchi and Kandatsu 1959). This monophosphonate is present both as a free molecule and incorporated in lipids as phospholipids, and in other macromolecules. It occurs in plants as well as in many animals species, mostly in membranes.

The biologic role of the monophosphonates is still unknown. One possibility is that they may make the molecule in which they are incorporated more resistant to enzymatic degradation. Possibly they also act as a phosphorus source in lower organisms. The synthesis of the C–P bond seems to be restricted to lower organisms such as bacteria, phytoplankton, protozoa, and invertebrates. The monophosphonates present in vertebrates come most probably from the diet or in cattle from rumen organisms as well (Smith 1983).

Monophosphonates have been used for a variety of purposes. One biologic application has been their use as analogs of natural phosphates for the elucidation of biochemical mechanisms. This property to act as analogs has also been made use of for chemotherapeutic purposes. Thus, certain phosphonates such as phosphonoformate and phosphonoacetate act as antimetabolites and are effective clinically against herpes and Epstein-Barr viruses by inhibiting DNA polymerase and therefore virus proliferation (Engel 1983). Certain streptomyces make a monophosphonate called fosfomycin which has antibiotic properties (Hendlin et al. 1969) and is used for this purpose in medicine. Other phosphonates act as insecticides, plant growth regulators, and chemical warfare agents on the basis of their inhibitory action on acetylcholinesterase (Hilderbrand 1983). Industrially, they have been used as adhesives, antioxidants, catalysts, corrosion inhibitors, flame and fire retardants, gelling agents, heat and light stabilizers, discoloration inhibitors, hydraulic fluid and fuel additives, ion exchange resins, lubricants, plasticizers, in photography, etc. (Drake and Calamari 1983).

History

Not only monophosphonates, but also bisphosphonates, have been known for some time in industry because of their various industrial applications, as water softeners (Drake and Calamari 1983) among others. This effect is due to their calcium-chelating property and their inhibition of calcium carbonate precipitation through crystal growth poisoning. However, our knowledge of their biologic characteristics dates from the last 20 years only. This has been derived from earlier studies on inorganic pyrophosphate (Fleisch and Russel 1970). We had found that biologic fluids such as plasma and urine contain compounds inhibiting calcium phosphate precipitation, and that part of this inhibitory activity is due to inorganic pyrophosphate, a compound which had not been described previously in these media (Fleisch and Neuman 1961; Fleisch and Bisaz 1962; Russell et al. 1971). Pyrophosphate was shown to impair the crystallization of calcium phosphate from solution (Fleisch and Neuman 1961) as well as the dissolution of these crystals (Fleisch et al. 1966). When given in vivo, pyrophosphate inhibits ectopic calcification induced by various means in tissues such as arteries, kidneys, and skin (Schibler et al. 1968). These effects are, however, present only when the compound is given parenterally, not when it is given orally. On the other hand, bone resorption is not influenced, possibly because pyrophosphate is hydrolyzed too quickly. On the basis of these results, it was suggested that pyrophosphate might be a physiologic regulator of calcification and perhaps also of decalcification in vivo, its local concentration being determined by the activity of local pyrophosphatases (Fleisch et al. 1966).

With the exception of the dental field, the therapeutic use of this compound in diseases where ectopic calcification or increased bone resorption occurs was, however, not likely to be successful, because of its failure to act when given orally, and because of its rapid hydrolysis when given parenterally. This prompted a search for analogs which would display similar physicochemical activity, but which would resist enzymatic hydrolysis and would therefore not be broken down metabolically. The bisphosphonates fulfilled these conditions.

Mode of Action

Physicochemical Effects

As was anticipated in view of the structural similarity between the bisphosphonates and pyrophosphate, the physicochemical effects of most of the bisphosphonates are very similar to those of pyrophosphate. Thus, many of the bisphosphonates inhibit the precipitation of calcium phosphate from clear solution, even at very low concentration (Fleisch et al. 1970; Meyer and Nancollas 1973), block the transformation of amorphous calcium phosphate into hydroxypatite (Francis 1969; Francis et al. 1969), and delay the aggregation of apatite crystals into larger clusters (Hansen et al. 1976). They also slow down the dissolution of these crystals (Fleisch et al. 1969; Russell et al. 1970). All these effects appear to be related to the marked affinity of these compounds for solid-phase calcium phosphate. Thus, they bind to the surface by chemisorption onto calcium (Jung et al. 1973), especially at screw dislocations and kink sites of growth, and then act as crystal poisons on both growth and dissolution. The binding is thought to be either bidentate, by means of the phosphate groups, or tridentate in the case of the hydroxybisphosphonates, the hydroxyl group making the third link (Barnett and Strickland 1979). Bisphosphonates also inhibit the formation (Fraser et al. 1972; Meyer et al. 1977) and the aggregation (Robertson et al. 1973) of calcium oxalate crystals.

Effect on Calcification In Vivo

Like pyrophosphate, bisphosphonates also inhibit calcification in vivo very efficiently. Thus, they prevent experimentally induced calcification of the arteries, kidneys, skin, and heart (Fleisch et al. 1970; Casey et al. 1972; Rosenblum et al. 1977) among others. In contrast to pyrophosphate, which acts only when given parenterally, they are also active when administered orally. Interestingly, in the arteries the decrease not only mineral deposition, but also the accumulation of cholesterol, elastin, and collagen (Hollander et al. 1978; Kramsch and Chan 1978). Bisphosphonates can also inhibit the calcification of bioprosthetic heart valves (Levy et al. 1985) and platelet deposition onto them (Devanjee et al. 1984), as well as the formation of experimental urinary stones (Fraser et al. 1972). Finally, topical administration leads to a decreased formation of dental calculus (Briner et al. 1971). Certain bisphosphonates, among others HEBP, inhibit not only ectopic calcification, but can in certain cases also inhibit ectopic ossification, when given systemically (Plasmans et al. 1978), or locally in slow-release form (Ahrengart and Lindgren 1986).

Bisphosphonates can, if administered in sufficient doses, also impair the mineralization of normal calcified tissues such as bone (Jowsey et al. 1970; King et al. 1971; Schenk et al. 1973), cartilage (Schenk et al. 1973), and dentin (Larsson 1974). This can lead to an impairment of fracture healing (Lenehan et al. 1985). The inhibition is eventually reversed after discontinuation of the drug (Flora et al. 1980). In growing animals, the radiologic picture resembles that induced by vitamin D deficiency. However, the two conditions vary histologically (Bisaz et al. 1975b), indicating that the mechanism of action leading to the inhibition is different. The doses required to induce the block of mineralization vary according to the bisphosphonate used, the animal species, the length of the treatment, and the route of administration. The effect on bone occurs at a lower dose than that on cartilage.

There is a close relationship between the ability of an individual bisphosphonate to inhibit the formation of calcium phosphate in vitro and its effectiveness on ectopic calcification in vivo (Fleisch et al. 1970; Shinoda et al. 1983), suggesting that the latter can be explained in terms of a physicochemical mechanism. The geminal bisphosphonates (P–C–P bond) are the most effective, although the activity varies from compound to compound. The vicinal bisphosphonates (P–C–C–P bond) are less effective or not effective and the monophosphonates (C–P bond) are not effective at all.

The mechanism of the inhibition of normal mineralization is at present not completely clear, although it is likely to be due to a physicochemical mechanism. All compounds tested so far which are effective in vivo are also good inhibitors in vitro (Trechsel et al. 1977). The opposite is, however, not true. Cl_2MBP displays relatively little inhibitory activity on bone mineralization in spite of its strong inhibition of crystal growth in vitro and of soft tissue calcification in vivo (Schenk et al. 1973). The explanation for this discrepancy is not yet clear. Differences in availability are a possibility.

Inhibition of Bone Resorption

The fact that bisphosphonates inhibit calcium phosphate crystal dissolution in vitro led us to hypothesize that these compounds might also act on bone resorption in vivo. The hypothesis proved correct, but the reason from which it was derived was not. Bisphosphonates proved to be very powerful inhibitors of bone resorption when tested in a variety of conditions, both in vitro and in vivo. In vitro, they block bone resorption induced by various means (Reynolds et al. 1972), as well as dissolution of bone particles by macrophages (Chambers 1980; Reitsma et al. 1982). In growing rats, they block the degradation of both bone and cartilage and thus arrest the remodeling of the metaphysis which becomes club-shaped and radiologically more dense than normal (Schenk et al. 1973; Reitsma et al. 1980). This effect is currently used as a model to study the potency of new compounds (Schenk et al. 1986). In the mouse, a similar effect has been found, leading to a picture similar to that seen in gray-lethal congenital osteopetrotic mice (Reynolds et al. 1973). The inhibition of endogenous bone resorption has also been documented by ^{45}Ca kinetic studies and by hydroxyproline excretion (Gasser et al. 1972).

Bisphosphonates also impair bone resorption induced by various agents. They blunt the effect of parathyroid hormone (Fleisch et al. 1969; Russell et al. 1970) as well as that of retinoids. They also prevent various types of osteoporisis, such as that induced by heparin (Haehnel et al. 1973), corticosteroids (Jee et al. 1981), by immobilization (Muehlbauer et al. 1971), and ovariectomy (Wink et al. 1985). Finally, they inhibit tumoral invasion of bone (Jung et al. 1984; Pollard and Luckert 1985; Radl et al. 1985), as well as various types of tumoral hypercalcemia (Johnson et al. 1982; Martodam et al. 1983). In the dental field, they prevent periodontal destruction in rice rats (Leonard et al. 1979).

The degree of activity of individual bisphosphonates varies greatly from compound to compound (Shinoda et al. 1983). If the aliphatic carbon backbone is lengthened, there is an increase in activity up to nine carbon atoms, but a decrease in activity occurs with additional length. Adding a hydroxyl group to the carbon atom at position 1 increases potency. Amino derivatives with an amino group at the end of the side chain are extremely active. Here again, the length of the side chain is very important, the highest activity being found with a length of the side chain is very important, the highest activity being found with a length of four carbons (4-amino-1-hydroxybutylidene-1,1-bisphosphonate AHBuBP), which is active at doses as low as 1 μg phosphorus per kilogram per day s.c. in the rat

(Schenk et al. 1986). Lately, a series of cyclic geminal bisphosphonates has been synthesized (Benedict et al. 1985a, b), some of them such as 2-(2-pyridinyl)ethylidenebisphosphonate being active at 1 µg phosphorus per kilogram per day s.c. (Bevan et al. 1985). Of the five bisphosphonates tested clinically, AHBuBP is the most potent in the rat, followed by AHPrBP and AHHexBP, then by Cl_2MBP, HEBP being the least effective (Schenk et al. 1986). It is therefore evident that the intensity of the effect is exquisitely dependent on the side chain. While the P–C–P structure is a prerequisite for the activity, it is not sufficient by itself. It is also of interest that there is no relationship at all between the intensity of the inhibition of mineralization and of the inhibition of resorption.

It was hoped that the decrease in resorption would be accompanied by a conspicuous increase in calcium balance and in the mineral content of bone. Although this is sometimes the case, especially in growing animals, this increase is in most cases smaller than predicted (Gasser et al. 1972). In addition, it is only transient (Reitsma et al. 1980), since after a certain time, bone formation decreases almost in parallel with the change in resorption, probably because of the well-known coupling between formation and resorption. The main effect is therefore a reduction of bone turnover. The greatest increase in retention has been found with Cl_2MBP, the aminobisphosphonates, and 1-hydroxypentylidene-1,1-bisphosphonate.

Originally, it was thought that, by analogy with what occurs in mineralization, the bisphosphonates would act on bone resorption through their inhibitory effect on calcium phosphate crystal dissolution. This proved, however, to be a wrong assumption. Indeed, no correlation has been found between the inhibition of bone resorption in vivo and the inhibition of crystal dissolution in vitro (Shinoda et al. 1983). Furthermore, bisphosphonates alter the morphology of osteoclasts both in vitro and when administered in vivo (Schenk et al. 1973; Miller and Jee 1979). Finally, the fact that extremely small amounts are acting in vivo also makes a physicochemical effect unlikely. Thus, it seems that the action in vivo is mediated through other mechanisms, most probably cellular.

Biochemical and Cellular Effects

A great number of different biochemical effects of bisphosphonates have been described. These effects vary greatly and can sometimes even go in opposite directions with different compounds, or with the same compound at different concentrations. At present, no clear picture of a structure-effect relationships has been ascertained. Some of the effects may be relevant to bone resorption. Certain bisphosphonates (especially Cl_2MBP and HEBP) reduce lactic acid production through decreased glycolysis both in intact calvaria (Morgan et al. 1973) and in isolated bone and cartilage cells (Fast et al. 1978). Conversely, however, other bisphosphonates, such as AHPrBP or long-chain bisphosphonates, increase lactic acid production, possibly because of a toxic action (Ende 1979; Shinoda et al. 1983). Various bisphosphonates, especially Cl_2MBP, inhibit certain lysosomal enzymes in vitro (Felix et al. 1976) and diminish their activity when added to cultured calvaria (Morgan et al. 1973; Delaissé et al. 1985) or when given in vivo

(Doty et al. 1972; Ende 1979). Certain bisphosphonates such as Cl_2MBP and HEBP inhibit prostaglandin synthesis by bone cells or calvaria, both when added in vitro and when given in vivo (Felix et al. 1981; Ohya et al. 1985). Finally, various bisphosphonates inhibit the multiplication of bone macrophages in vitro, even at very low concentrations (Cecchini et al. 1987). Furthermore, they show cytotoxic and migration inhibitory effects on peritoneal macrophages (Stevenson and Stevenson 1986). Thus, macrophages seem to be specially sensitive to bisphosphonates.

Numerous additional cellular actions have been described for individual bisphosphonates. These include: an increase of fatty acid oxidation (Felix and Fleisch 1981) and amino oxidation (Ende 1979); a stimulation of the citric acid cycle (Ende 1979); an increase in cellular content of glycogen (Felix et al. 1980); an increase in the production of alkaline phosphatase (Felix and Fleisch 1979); an increase in the biosynthesis of bone and cartilage collagen (Guenther et al. 1981a, b), possibly by impaired intracellular collagenolysis (Gallagher et al. 1982); an impairment of dentin and cementum formation (Beertsen et al. 1985); an increase in the synthesis of proteoglycans in vitro (Guenther et al. 1979), but a decrease when administered in vivo (Larrson 1976); a reduction in the release of calcium from kidney mitochondria in vitro (Guilland et al. 1974) and an increase in calcium of mitochondria in vivo (Plasmans et al. 1980); contradictory effects on cAMP production (Pilczyk et al. 1972; Gebauer et al. 1976); a decrease or an increase in cellular multiplication (Fast et al. 1978; Evêquoz et al. 1985); an inhibition of amebal phosphofructokinase, which raised the possibility of their use in amebiasis (Eubank and Reeves 1982); in the case of certain thiobisphosphonates an inhibition of interleukin-1-induced enzymes release take of over (Edmonds-Alt et al. 1985); an inhibition of the action of mitogens on mononuclear function and on the lymphoblastic response (De Vries et al. 1982); and an inhibition of the influence of antilymphocyte serum on T-lymphocytes (Zernov et al. 1979).

These findings suggest that bisphosphonates enter mammalian cells. This has been confirmed by studies in vitro, both for HEBP and Cl_2MBP (Fast et al. 1978). The cellular uptake was mostly in the cytosol and the concentration expressed in terms of cellular water can be severalfold higher than in the medium, indicating that the bisphosphonates are accumulating within specific cellular compartments (Felix et al. 1984). Cells with phagocytic properties can also take up bisphosphonates, with especial avidity if the compounds are bound to apatite crystals (Chambers 1980), or when they are encapsulated into liposomes, in which case they are also taken up in vivo by the spleen (Van Rooijen et al. 1985).

Mode of Action in the Inhibition of Bone Resorption

From this variety of biochemical and cellular effects, some may be candidates to play a role in the inhibition of bone resorption. The decrease in lactic acid production may be relevant, since it is thought that acid production plays an important role in crystal dissolution. The same might be true for the inhibition of lysosomal enzymes, as these are thought to be important in matrix degradation, and for the inhibition of the synthesis of prostaglandins, powerful bone resorbers. Since osteoclasts originate from the monocyte macrophage system, the inhibitory effect on the multiplication of bone macrophages might lead to a decrease in osteoclast recruitment. The initial hypothesis of a physicochemical effect cannot be rejected completely either. Finally, some compounds, especially at high doses, may act through a toxic effect on the relevant cells.

Unfortunately, studies performed up to now with various bisphosphonates have not shown a correlation between any of these biologic effects and the inhibition of bone resorption in vivo (Shinoda et al. 1983). Thus, none of these mechanisms is the *only* explanation for the inhibition of bone resorption, although it cannot be ruled out that some or all of them may contribute and that bisphosphonates have various modes of action. Recent results suggest that certain bisphosphonates, such as Cl_2MBP, lead to a decrease of osteoclasts, while others, such as the aminobisphosphonates, induce an increased number of osteoclasts, this in spite of the fact that bone resorption is blocked (Stutzer et al. 1987b).

In view of the large array of cellular effects of bisphosphonates, it might be found surprising that they act almost exclusively on calcified tissues. This selectivity probably stems from the strong affinity of these compounds for calcium phosphate which allows them to be cleared very rapidly from blood and to be incorporated into calcified tissues, especially bone (Jung et al. 1973; Bisaz et al. 1978). Whenever the latter is resorbed, the compounds will be released into the surrounding solution, either in free form or bound onto the surface of apatite crystals. They can thus reach high local concentration in the vicinity of the resorbing cells and be taken up by these, either as free compounds or with the crystals. This may explain why one administration of bisphosphonates can be active for long periods, both in animals (Stutzer et al. 1987a) and in humans. It now appears that the role of the P–C–P moiety of the bisphosphonates is mainly to confer on them their affinity for the mineralized tissues and thus target the effect on these. On the other hand, their cellular effect seems to be conferred by the whole molecule, and is thus dependent on the structure of the side chains. This opens the exciting possibility of the synthesis of new compounds with stronger antiresorbing effects.

Other Effects

Besides the effects on mineralized tissues, some other actions have been described in vivo, mostly, however, after large doses. A few concefn the immune system. A decrease in the formation of antibody-secreting cells in response to immunization and an impaired delayed and immediate hypersensitivity has been found (Komissarenko et al. 1977). Cl_2MBP given to newborn mice leads to atrophy of the thymus (Milhaud et al. 1983), to the disappearance of certain thymus-dependent macrophages (Labat et al. 1983), of natural killer cells (Labat et al. 1984), and to a diminution of the response of T-lymphocytes to mitogens (Milhaud et al. 1983). It is interesting that the latter changes have also been found in osteopetrotic mice. However, the doses of bisphosphonates which lead to these changes are very high, so that it is not clear if the latter are relevant to the effects of the compounds on bone. In this line it is also of interest that a thiobisphosphonate has been found to inhibit passive cutaneous anaphylaxis (Barbier et al. 1985) and that Cl_2MBP,

HEBP, and a thiobisphosphonate inhibit some of the changes seen in adjuvant-induces polyarthritis (Francis et al. 1972; Flora 1979; Barbier et al. 1986). Various bisphosphonates also inhibit the 1,25-dihydroxy vitamin D-induced increase in plasma osteocalcin in rats (Stronski et al. 1985).

Other effects of bisphosphonates are probably secondary to their skeletal action. Large doses of HEBP decrease the intestinal absorption of calcium (Bonjour et al. 1973) because of a decrease in the formation of 1,25-dihydroxy vitamin D_3 (Hill et al. 1973; Baxter et al. 1974), while low doses induce an increase in the hormone formation (Guilland et al. 1975). These changes are likely to be due to an indirect homeostatic mechanism aimed at adapting intestinal calcium absorption to the needs of the organism. The large doses act via their inhibition of mineralization, while with the smaller doses, where no such inhibition of calcification occurs, the triggering mechanism is the decreased bone resorption. A similar indirect mechanism is probably also the cause of the decreased capacity of the kidney to reabsorb phosphate found in the rat under HEBP treatment (Bonjour et al. 1978).

Pharmacokinetics

Bisphosphonates are synthetic compounds which have not yet been found to occur naturally in animals or humans. No enzymes able to cleave the P–C–P bond have yet been described. According to our current knowledge, the administered bisphosphonates are absorbed, stored, and excreted unaltered in animals. Thus, bisphosphonates appear to be nonbiodegradable, both in animals and in solution (Steber and Wierich 1986). Most of the pharmacokinetic data on bisphosphonates have been obtained with HEBP or Cl_2MBP. The intestinal absorption lies between 1% and 10% of an oral dose, is generally higher in the young, higher when ingestion increases, and shows a great inter- and intraspecies variation (Michael et al. 1972; Recker and Saville 1973; Gural 1975). In humans, absorption is 1%–9% for HEBP (Fogelman et al. 1986), and 1%–2% for Cl_2MBP (Yakatan et al. 1982). Absorption occurs, at least in the rat, mostly in the small intestine (Wasserman et al. 1973) and is diminished by the presence of calcium (see Francis and Martodam 1983). This is the reason why bisphosphonates have always to be given to humans before meals and never together with milk products. The absorption is inversely related to the size of the compounds, some of the large polyphosphonates being virtually nonabsorbable (Anbar et al. 1973).

Between 20% and 50% of the absorbed HEBP is localized to bone, the remainder being rapidly excreted in the urine (Michael et al. 1972). The excreted part is somewhat larger for Cl_2MBP (Conrad and Lee 1981). The renal clearance of HEBP and Cl_2MBP exceeds that of inulin, suggesting the presence of a secretory pathway (Troehler et al. 1975). Sometimes, bisphosphonates can deposit in other organs such as the liver (Wingen and Schmaehl 1975). This might be due to the formation of particles after too rapid intravenous injection, which are then phagocytosed by the reticuloendothelial system.

The half-life of circulating bisphosphonates is only of the order of minutes, the rate of entry into bone being very fast, similar to that of calcium and phosphate (Bisaz et al. 1978; Conrad and Lee 1981; Yakatan et al. 1982). Therefore, soft tissues will be exposed to these compounds for only short periods. On the other hand, the half-time of the skeletal retention is long and depends on the turnover rate of the skeleton itself.

Toxicology

Toxicologic animal studies reported to date deals almost exclusively with HEBP and Cl_2MBP. Acute, subacute, and chronic administration in several animal species have revealed little toxicity. Teratogenic, mitogenic, and carcinogenic tests were negative (Nolen and Buehler 1971; Nixon et al. 1972). The acute toxicity appears to be due to the formation of complexes with calcium, leading to hypocalcemia. Whenm the compound is administered intravenously, it varies with the speed of infusion (Francis and Slough 1984). The first chronic side effect is the appearance of fractures at about 0.15 mg phosphorus per kilogram s.c. for HEBP and 0,7 mg phosphorus per kilogram. s.c. for Cl_2MBP (Flora et al. 1980). With HEBP at 0.6 mg phosphorus per kilogram an inhibition of mineralization occurs. This is not seen with Cl_2MBP at doses at high as 7 mg phosphorus per kilogram (Flora et al. 1980). At higher doses, renal lesions appear. Furthermore, inflammatory gastric lesions (even when the compounds are given parenterally) as well as pulmonary lesions have been reported. However, it must be stressed that these results cannot necessarily be extrapolated to other bisphosphonates. Indeed, in our experience, toxicity, both in culture and in vivo, varies greatly from one compound to another, so that great caution has to be applied when using new compounds clinically.

Drug Interactions

No interactions have been described up to now.

Clinical Use

The studies described have led to trials of various bisphosphonates in human diseases. Clinical applications have focused upon three main areas: (a) use as skeletal markers in the form of ^{99m}Tc derivatives for diagnostic purposes in nuclear medicine; (b) therapeutic use in patients with ectopic calcification and ossification; and (c) therapeutic use in patients with increased bone destruction. Only the therapeutic aspects will be discussed here, the application in scintigraphy being beyond the scope of this chapter. Until now, three bisphosphonates, namely HEBP, Cl_2MBP, and AHPrBP, have been investigated on a larger scale in humans. First results have been reported with AHBuBP and AHHexBP. Only HEBP and Cl_2MBP are on the market for clinical use. In the dental field, another bisphosphonate, azacycloheptylidene-2,2-bisphosphonate, is on sale in a toothpaste.

Ectopic Calcification and Ossification

Based on the preventive effect of bisphosphonates, especially HEBP, on ectopic calcifications and ectopic ossifications in animals, it was hoped that a similar effect would be found in human diseases involving abnormal mineralization. Generally speaking, the results are ambiguous in ectopic calcification, but encouraging in ectopic ossification.

Soft Tissue Calcification

HEBP has been given in some cases of scleroderma (Metzger et al. 1974; Rabens and Bethune 1975), dermatomyositis (Metzger et al. 1974; Steiner et al. 1974), and calcinosis universalis (Cram et al. 1971). Efficacy is uncertain since these disorders often show spontaneous remissions.

Urolithiasis

The hope that the inhibitory effect on crystal growth and aggregation of both calcium phosphate and calcium oxalate would be useful for the prevention of urinary stones has not been fulfilled, at least with HEBP. Although pilot studies showed a certain effect in chronic stone formers (Baumann et al. 1978; Bone et al. 1979), the necessary dose to obtain inhibition of crystal growth in urine is high, about 1600 mg/day orally (Ohata and Pak 1974; Baumann et al. 1978), so that it will also induce skeletal effects. Furthermore, the clinical benefit is uncertain, other large-scale studies having failed to show efficacy. Bisphosphonates cannot therefore be recommended for use in urolithiasis.

Dental Calculus

Many investigations have shown that topical application of HEBP diminishes the development of dental calculus (Muehlemann et al. 1970; Sturzenberger et al. 1971). Azacycloheptylidene-2,2-bisphosphonate is added to a toothpaste which has been marketed in various countries.

Fibrodysplasia Ossificans Progressiva

This disease, also called myositis ossificans progressiva, is the first in which a bisphosphonate, HEBP, has been investigated in humans (Bassett et al. 1969). Despite a series of further investigations (Geho and Whiteside 1973; Reiner et al. 1980), it remains to be established whether this drug is really active in decreasing ectopic bone formation. It appears that some retardation in the evolution of the disease can occur, but that a complete standstill is rarely obtained. Already formed lesions are not influenced. Despite this uncertainty, in view of the outcome of the disease and the lack of alternative treatment, the use of HEBP in a dosage of 20 mg kg^{-1} day^{-1} seems advisable. Since effective doses also inhibit mineralization of normal bone and can, at least in children, lead to rickets (Reiner et al. 1980), the drug should not be given for longer than 3 months, but better for shorter periods of a few weeks, and only when a new exacerbation occurs.

Other Heterotopic Ossifications

Results seem more encouraging with other types of heterotopic ossifications. HEBP has been found to diminish the appearance of ossifications in patients with spinal cord injury (Finerman and Stover 1981), after cranial trauma (Spielman et al. 1983), and after total hip replacement (Slooff et al. 1974; Finerman and Stover 1981). In the latter, although ectopic bone formation reappears, at least partially, after discontinuation of the drug, the mobility of the hip seems nevertheless to be improved in the HEBP-treated patients. Recently, however, these results have been questioned (Thomas and Amstutz 1985).

Although its efficacy is not absolutely ascertained, it seems nevertheless justifiable to administer HEBP preventively, especiall to those patients who are particularly liable to develop ectopic ossifications, for example, patients who requiere a second operation after total hip replacement because of ossifications after the first intervention. The daily oral dosage lies between 800 and 1600 mg, given for 3 months and starting just before the operation. A longer treatment should not be given because of the inhibition of normal mineralization.

Abnormally Increased Bone Resorption

Paget's Disease

The main clinical use of bisphosphonates today is in patients with Paget's disease, a condition characterized by an increased skeletal turnover. All three bisphosphonates, HEBP, Cl_2MP, and AHPrBP, are effective in this disease in decreasing turnover, the largest number of investigations having been performed with HEBP. HEBP decreases both serum alkaline phosphatase, an index of bone formation, as well as urinary hydroxyproline excretion, an index of bone destruction (Smith et al. 1971; Altman et al. 1973; Russell et al. 1974; De Vries and Bijvoet 1974). The effect on hydroxyproline usually precedes that on alkaline phosphatase, suggesting that the primary effect of the bisphosphonate is on bone resorption, the effect on bone formation being possibly secondary to the coupling between the two processes. The action of HEBP on bone turnover is also illustrated by ^{45}Ca kinetic studies (Guncaga et al. 1974; De Vries and Bijvoet 1974) and by morphological studies (Russell et al. 1974; Guncaga et al. 1974; De Vries and Bijvoet 1974; Meunier et al. 1975). It is interesting that the bone formed under treatment is lamellar, in contrast to the woven bon typical of this disease. However, HEBP does not affect the virus-induced measles nucleocapsid-like inclusions in the nuclei of the osteoclasts, nor the measles-type viral antigens in the osteoclasts (Basle et al. 1984). HEBP decreases the elevated cardiac output (Henley et al. 1979) and the subjective symptoms such as bone pain (Altman et al. 1973; Meunier et al. 1975). On the other hand, no improvement in the X-ray picture can be obtained (De Vries and Bijvoet 1974; Canfield et al. 1977). In fact, in certain cases, the drug induces the appearance of radiolucent areas (Nagant De Deuxchaisnes et al. 1979), which probably reflect locations of impaired mineralization.

Indeed, oral doses between 800 and 1600 mg have been shown to induce an inhibition of mineralization of both pagetic and normal bone (Russell et al. 1974; Guncaga et al. 1974; De Vries and Bijvoet 1974; Meunier et al. 1975). This inhibition is reversible when the treatment is stopped. Oral doses of 400 mg do not lead to this generalized inhibition of mineralization, but can occasionally produce focal osteomalacia (Boyce et al. 1984). Fractures have been described under HEBP therapy. However, fractures are also more frequent in untreated patients, so that the role of treatment is difficult to assess (Johnston et al. 1983). Since the margin between the dose of HEBP which inhibits resorption and that which inhibits mineralization is small, and since intestinal absorption of the compound is not only small, but very variable from patient to patient, the optimal dosage is difficult to define. The generally recommended dose is either 1600 mg orally for maximally 3 months or 800 mg orally for 6 months to 1 year. Other modes of oral treatment such as intermittent dosage (Siris et al. 1980a) or an association with calcitonin have not been investigated well enough yet. It has been shown that treatment for 1 month with 1600 mg/day is as effective as treatment for 6 months with the same dose, and more effective than treatment for 6 months with 400 mg/day (Preston et al. 1986).

Also, Cl_2MBP has been found to be very active in decreasing bone turnover in Paget's disease, although the clinical experience is much smaller than for HEBP. Oral daily doses between 800 and 1600 mg decrease both urinary hydroxyproline and serum alkaline phosphatase (Meunier et al. 1979; Douglas et al. 1980). In analogy to what was found in animals, these doses of Cl_2MBP induce, contrary to HEBP, no inhibition of bone mineralization (Meunier et al. 1979). Treatment for 1 month (Chapuy et al. 1983) is as effective as treatment for 6 months. This is also true for 5 days intravenous administration of 300 mg/day (Yates et al. 1985), a treatment which produces a maximal effect on urinary hydroxyproline after 4-5 days.

The third bisphosphonate investigated in Paget's disease is AHPrBP. As in animals, this is the most active of the three compounds and is effective at an oral daily dose of 200-1600 mg. Again, both parameters of bone turnover, urinary hydroxyproline and serum alkaline phosphatase, are decreased (Frijlink et al. 1979; Heynen et al. 1982). All the bisphosphonates maintain their action months and even years after discontinuation of the therapy (Russell et al. 1974; Siris et al. 1980a; Chapuy et al. 1983), in contrast to calcitonin, which is active only as long as it is administered.

Primary Hyperparathyroidism

While the oral administration of HEBP has been found ineffective in this condition (Kaplan et al. 1977), Cl_2MBP at oral daily doses between 1200 and 3200 mg decreases the degree of hypercalcemia, the level of serum alkaline phosphatase, and the urinary excretion of hydroxyproline and calcium (Douglas et al. 1980; Shane et al. 1981).

Hypercalcemia of Malignancy and Tumoral Bone Destruction

A Variety of tumors can produce bone destruction and hypercalcemia. The mechanism involves either the production of humoral osteolytic cytokines by a tumor situated outside the bone, or the local destruction of the bone by the tumor in situ. Both types respond to bisphosphonates (see Garattini 1985). HEBP has been found to be of little use when given orally, but to lead to a rapid decrease in calcemia and often to a normalization within 3–4 days when given intravenously at a daily dose of around 500 mg (Jung 1982; Ryzen et al. 1985).

Cl_2MBP, on the other hand, displays activity on a variety of tumors when given orally at a dose between 1600 and 3200 mg/day (Chapuy et al. 1980; Siris et al. 1980b, 1983). Calcemia can be restored to normal and calciuria is decreased dramatically. Intravenous administration of 120–1200 mg decreases calcemia as soon as 2 days after starting the treatment, normal values being obtained within 5–7 days (Jung 1982; Siris et al. 1980b; Jacobs et al. 1981). Of great clinical interest is the finding that the bisphosphonate also inhibitis the development of new metastases (Elomaa et al. 1983). Also, AHPrBP is effective in various tumors and again it appears to be the most active of the three. Doses of 300–1500 mg orally (Van Breukelen et al. 1979, 1982) and 1.6–24 mg intravenously (Sleeboom et al. 1983) are effective. Even a single administration appears to be effective (Thiébaud et al. 1986).

Osteoporosis

There have been only a few studies so far using bisphosphonates in patients with osteoporosis. HEBP did not significantly improve calcium balance in senile osteoporosis, although bone turnover was cut down by about 50% (Heaney and Saville 1976). However, the dosage used was too high, at a level which induces inhibition of mineralization, which could have masked a positive effect. No effect on calcium balance was found either during bed rest, a condition which is associated with enhanced skeletal turnover and negative calcium balance (Lockwood et al. 1975). Recently, however, it has been reported that discontinuous oral administration of 400 mg/day for 2 weeks every 15 weeks over a period of 2 years leads to a 6% increase of trabecular bone in the spine of postmenopausal women, while controls lost 5% (Storm et al. 1987). Cl_2MBP at an oral dose of 1600 mg/day partially prevented the osteoporosis of immobilization in paraplegic patients (Minaire et al. 1981). This result suggests that bisphosphonates might be used in the future for the prevention of at least high turnover osteoporosis.

Side Effects

As in animals, studies in humans have revealed few important side effects. The first and major complication under HEBP therapy is the inhibition of normal skeletal mineralization. This effect appears at daily oral doses between 800 and 1600 mg (Russell et al. 1974; Jowsey et al. 1971; Guncaga et al. 1974; De Vries and Bijvoet 1974). Fractures have occurred in children (Reiner et al. 1980) and possibly also in adults, although in the latter the cause-effect relation has not yet been proven with certainty (Johnston et al. 1983). In children, long-term treatment at an oral dosage of 20 mg/kg may induce proximal muscular weakness leading to an abnormal gait, similar to that seen in rickets (Reiner et al. 1980). HEBP also causes a conspicuous rise in plasma phosphate, often to high levels, both in healthy persons and in patients. The change is associated with an increase in renal tubular reabsorption of phosphate (Recker et al. 1973; Walton et al. 1975). It seems that hyperphosphatemia shows a correlation with the degree of inhibition of bone mineralization, but the reason for this correlation is as yet unclear. Caution must be taken with the intravenous administration of HEBP, since a rapid injection has led to renal failure (Bounameaux et al. 1983), possibly because of the precipitation of calcium bisphosphonate or the formation of calcium bisphosphonate aggregates in the blood.

No proven side effects have been described as yet for Cl_2MBP. Contrary to HEBP, this compound does not inhibit mineralization of bone and does not induce hyperphosphatemia. In the course of the clinical evaluation of this compound, some of the treated patients have developed acute leukemia. However, further evaluation cast doubs that the disease was induced by the drug so that it is quite possible that this finding was fortuitous.

Finally, AHPrBP does not induce an inhibition of bone mineralization at doses active on bone resorption. This compound does not lead at this dosage to an increase in plasma phosphate. On the other hand, AHPrBP induces during the first few days a transient increase in temperature and a leukopenia (Bijvoet et al. 1980). Furthermore, this substance appears to lead to alterations of the oral and digestive mucosa under certain circumstances when given orally.

Future Prospects

The bisphosphonates present a most interesting new development in the field of the treatment of bone diseases. It is probable that this is only the beginning of a new area of therapy. Indeed, since the effects vary greatly from one bisphosphonate to another, it is quite possible that new bisphosphonates may be synthesized which are superior to those known up to now. It will be especially desirable to develop compounds with a greater margin between the dose inhibiting bone resorption and that inhibiting mineralization. For such a development it would be advantageous to know the mechanisms of action and to be in possession of a structure-effect relationship for the compounds. It might also be possible in future to find bisphosphonates which act more on ectopic calcification than on normal mineralization. Recent results suggest that certain bisphosphonates might also be active in rheumatic diseases. Finally, with the exception of ^{99m}Tc in nuclear medicine, the possible use of bisphosphonates as carriers of drugs acting on the skeleton has not been examined at all and may also be an interesting development.

Summary

The geminal bisphosphonates are characterized by a PCP bond and are therefore analogs of pyrophosphate. They bind strongly to hydroxyapatite crystals and in vitro inhibit both crystal formation and dissolution. In vivo they inhibit soft tissue calcification and when given in large amounts also normal calcification. This effect is due to the inhibition of calcium phosphate crystal growth.

Furthermore, the bisphosphonates are very potent inhibitors of bone resorption. The mechanism(s) of action is not yet known but is likely to be at a cellular level. The extent of the biological activity of each compound depends on the specific chemical structure, so that each individual bisphosphonate must be considered as a separate compound. The only common characteristic is the PCP group, which gives the compound its high affinity to bone. The individual effects, however, are determined by the side groups on the carbon atom. This opens interesting possibilities for the development of new compounds.

No bisphosphonate analyzed so far can be degraded in vivo; all are either deposited in the skeleton, where they remain for years until the bone is destroyed, or are excreted in the urine. The high affinity for bone explains the specificity of the compounds for bone and the fact that they have relatively few nonosseous effects.

Bisphosphonates are used in man to inhibit ectopic calcification, including dental tartar and ectopic ossification. Furthermore, they are used to inhibit bone resorption, especially in diseases such as Paget's disease and tumoral osteolysis. Finally, when linked to ^{99n}Tc, bisphosphonates are employed as bone scanning agents.

References

Ahrengart L, Lindgren U (1986) Prevention of ectopic bone formation by local application of ethane-1-hydroxy-1,1-diphosphonate (EHDP): an experimental study in rabbits. J Orthop Res 4: 18–26

Altmann RD, Johnston CC, Khairi MRA, Wellman H, Serafini AN, Sankey RR (1973) Influence of disodium etidronate on clinical and laboratory manifestations of Paget's disease of bone (osteitis deformans). N Engl J Med 289: 1379–1384

Anbar M, Newell GW, St John GA (1973) Fate and toxicity of orally administered polyethylene polyphosphonates. Food Cosmetics Tox 11: 1001–1010

Barbier A, Brelière JC, Paul RP, Roncucci R (1985) Comparative study of etidronate and SR 41319, a new diphosphonate, on passive cutaneous anaphylaxis and phospholipase A_2 activity. Agents Actions 16: 41–42

Barbier A, Brelière JC, Remandet B, Roncucci R (1986) Studies on the chronic phase of adjuvant arthritis: effect of SR 41319, a new diphosphonate. Ann Rheum Dis 45: 67–74

Barnett BL, Stickland LC (1979) Structure of disodium dihydrogen 1-hydroxyethylidenediphosphonate tetrahydrate: a bone growth regulator. Acta Crystall ogr B35: 1212–1214

Basle MF, Rebel A, Renier JC, Audran M, Filmon R, Malkani K (1984) Bone tissue in Paget's disease treated by ethane-1-hydroxy-1,1 diphosphonate (EHDP). Clin Orthop Rel Res 184: 281-288

Bassett CAL, Donath A, Macagno F, Preisig R, Fleisch H, Francis MD (1969) Diphosphonates in the treatment of myositis ossificans. Lancet 2: 845

Baumann JM, Bisaz S, Fleisch H, Wacker M (1978) Biochemical and clinical effects of ethane-1-hydroxy-1,1-diphosphonate on calcium nephrolithiasis. Clin Sci Mol Med 54: 509-516

Baxter LA, DeLuca HF, Bonjour JP, Fleisch H (1974) Inhibition of vitamin D metabolism by ethane-1-hydroxy-1,1-diphosphonate. Arch Biochem Biophys 164: 655-662

Beertsen W, Niehof A, Everts V (1985) Effects of 1-hydroxyethylidene-1,1-bisphosphonate (HEBP) on the formation of dentin and the periodontal attachment apparatus in the mouse. Am J Anat 174: 83-103

Benedict JJ, Degenhardt CR, Perkins CM, Johnson KY, Bevan JA, Olson HM (1985a) Cyclic geminal bis(phosphonates) as inhibitors of bone resorption. Calcif Tissue Int 38 [Suppl]: S31

Benedict JJ, Johnson KY, Bevan JA, Perkins CM (1985b) A structure/activity study of nitrogen heterocycle containing bis(phosphonates) as bone resorption inhibiting agents. Calcif Tissue Int 38 [Suppl]: S31

Bevan JA, Johnson KY, Slough C, Benedict J, Fleisch H, Black J (1985) Skeletal effects of 2-(2-pyridinyl)-ethylidene-bis(phosphonate) in acute and subchronic rat studies. Calcif Tissue Int 38 [Suppl]: S31

Bijvoet OLM, Frijlink WB, Jie K, Linden H van der, Meijer CJLM, Mulder H, Paassen HC van, Reitsma PH, Velde J te, Vries E de, Wey JP van der (1980) APD in Paget's disease of bone. Role of the mononuclear phagocyte system? Arthritis Rheum 23: 1193-1204

Bisaz S, Felix R, Fleisch H (1975a) Quantitative determination of ethane-1-hydroxy-1,1-diphosphonate in urine and plasma. Clin Chim Acta 65: 299-307

Bisaz S, Schenk R, Kunin AS, Russell RGG, Mühlbauer R, Fleisch H (1975b) The comparative effects of vitamin D deficiency and ethane-1-hydroxy-1,1-diphosphonate administration on the histology and glycolysis of chick epiphyseal and articular cartilage. Calcif Tissue Res 19:139-152

Bisaz S, Jung A, Fleisch H (1978) Uptake by bone of pyrophosphate, diphosphonates and their technetium derivatives. Clin Sci Mol Med 54: 265-272

Blaser B, Worms KH, Germscheid HG, Wollmann K (1971) Ueber 1-Hydroxyalkan-1,1-diphosphonsäuren. Z Anorg Allg Chem 381: 247-259

Bone HG, Zerwekh JE, Britton F, Pak CYC (1979) Treatment of calcium urolithiasis with diphosphonate: efficacy and hazards. J Urol 121: 568-571

Bonjour JP, Russell RGG, Morgan DB, Fleisch H (1973) Intestinal calcium absorption, Ca-binding protein, and Ca-ATPase in diphosphonate-treated rats. Am J Physiol 224: 1011-1017

Bonjour JP, Tröhler U, Preston C, Fleisch H (1978) Parathyroid hormone and renal handling of Pi: effect of dietary Pi and diphosphonates. Am J Physiol 234: F487-F505

Bounameaux HM, Schifferli J, Montani JP, Jung A, Chatelanat F (1983) Renal failure associated with intravenous diphosphonate. Lancet 1: 471

Boyce BF, Fogelman I, Ralston S, Smith L, Johnston E, Boyle IT (1984) Focal osteomalacia due to low-dose diphosphonate therapy in Paget's disease. Lancet 1: 821-824

Briner WW, Francis MD, Widder JS (1971) The control of dental calculus in experimental animals. Int Dent J 21: 61-73

Canfield R, Rosner W, Skinner J, McWorther J, Resnick L, Feldman F, Kammerman S, Ryan K, Kunigonis M, Bohne W (1977) Diphosphonate therapy of Paget's disease of bone. J Clin Endocrinol Metab 44: 96-106

Casey PA, Casey G, Fleisch H, Russell RGG (1972) The effect of polyphloretin phosphate, polyestradiol phosphate, a diphosphonate and a polyphosphate on calcification induced by dihydrotachysterol in skin, aorta and kidney of rats. Experientia 28: 137-138

Cecchini M, Felix R, Cooper PH, Fleisch H (1987) Effect of bisphosphonates on proliferation and viability of mouse bone marrow-derived macrophages. J Bone Min Res 2: 135: 142

Chambers TJ (1980) Diphosphonates inhibit bone resorption by macrophages in vitro. J Pathol 132: 255-262

Chapuy MC, Meunier PJ, Alexandre CM, Vignon EP (1980) Effects of disodium dichloromethylene diphosphonate on hypercalcemia produced by bone metastases. J Clin Invest 65: 1243-1247

Chapuy MC, Charhon SA, Meunier PJ (1983) Sustained biochemical effects of short treatment of Paget's disease of bone with dichloromethylene diphosphonate. Metab Bone Dis Rel Res 4: 325-328

Chester TL, Lewis EC, Benedict JJ, Sunberg RJ, Tettenhorst WC (1981) Determination of (dichloromethylene)diphosphonate in physiological fluids by ion-exchange chromatography with phosphorus-selective detection. J Chromatogr Sci 225: 17-25

Conrad KA, Lee SM (1981) Clodronate kinetics and dynamics. Clin Pharmacol Ther 30: 114-120

Cram RL, Barmada R, Geho WB, Ray RD (1971) Diphosphonate treatment of calcinosis universalis. N Engl J Med 285: 1012-1013

Curry JD, Nicholson DA (1972) Oligophosphonates. In: Griffith J, Grayson M (eds) Topics in phosphorus chemistry, vol 7. Wiley, New York, p 37

Delaissé J-M, Eeckhout Y, Vaes G (1985) Biphosphonates and bone resorption: effects on collagenase and lysosomal enzyme excretion. Life Sci 37: 2291-2296

De Vries HR, Bijvoet OLM (1974) Results of prolonged treatment of Paget's disease of bone with disodium ethane-1-hydroxy-1,1-diphosphonate (EHDP). Neth J Med 17: 281-298

De Vries E, Weij JP van der, Veen CJP v d, Paassen HC van, Jager MJ, Sleeboom HP, Bijvoet OLM, Cats A (1982) In vitro effect of (3-amino-1-hydroxypropylidene)-1,1-bisphosphonic acid (APD) on the function of mununuclear phagocytes in lymphocyte proliferation. Immunology 47: 157-163

Dewanjee MK, Didisheim P, Kaye MP, Solis E, Zollman PE, Francis MD, Torianni M, Trastek VS, Tago M, Edwards WD (1984) Platlet deposition on and calcification of bovine pericardial valve. Eur Heart J 5 [Suppl D]: 1-5

Doty SB, Jones R, Finerman GA (1972) Diphosphonate influence on bone cell structure and lysosomal activity. J Bone Joint Surg 54: 1128-1129

Douglas DL, Russell RGG, Preston CJ, Prenton MA, Duckworth T, Kanis JA, Preston FE, Woodhead JS (1980) Effect of dichloromethylene diphosphonate in Paget's disease of bone and in hypercalcaemia due to primary hyperparathyroidism or malignant disease. Lancet 1: 1043-1047

Drake GL, Calamari TA (1983) Industrial uses of phosphonates. In: Hilderbrand RL (ed) The role of phosphonates in living systems. CRC, Boca Raton, p 171

Elomaa I, Blomqvist C, Gröhn P, Porkka L, Kairento AL, Selander K, Lamberg-Allardt C, Holmström T (1983) Long-term controlled trial with diphosphonate in patients with osteolytic bone metastases. Lancet 1: 146-149

Emonds-Alt X, Brelière J-C, Roncucci R (1985) Effects of 1-hydroxyethylidene-1,1 bisphosphonate and (chloro-4 phenyl) thiomethylene bisphosphonic acid (SR 41319) on the mononuclear cell factor-mediated release of neutral proteinases by articular chondrocytes and synovial cells. Biochem Pharmacol 34: 4043-4049

Ende JJ (1979) Effects of some diphosphonates on the metabolism of bone in vivo and in vitro. Thesis, University of Leiden

Engel R (1983) Phosphonic acids and phosphonates as antimetabolites. In: Hilderbrand RL (ed) The role of phosphonates in living systems. CRC, Boca Raton, p 97

Eubank WB, Reeves RE (1982) Analog inhibitors for the pyrophosphate-dependent phosphofructokinase of Entamoeba histolytica and their effect of culture growth. J Parasitol 68: 599-602

Evêquoz V, Trechsel U, Fleisch H (1985) Effect of bisphosphonates on production of interleukin 1-like activity by macrophages and its effect on rabbit chondrocytes. Bone 6: 439–444
Fast DK, Felix R, Dowse C, Neumann WF, Fleisch H (1978) The effects of diphosphonates on the growth and glycolysis of connective-tissue cells in culture. Biochem J 172: 97–107
Felix R, Fleisch H (1979) Increase in alkaline phosphatase activity in calvaria cells cultured with diphosphonates. Biochem J 183: 73–81
Felix R, Fleisch H (1981) Increase in fatty acid oxidation in calvaria cells cultured with diphosphonates. Biochem J 196: 237–245
Felix R, Russell RGG, Fleisch H (1976) The effect of several diphosphonates on acid phosphohydrolases and other lysosomal enzymes. Biochim Biophys Acta 429: 429–438
Felix R, Fast DK, Sallis JD, Fleisch H (1980) Effect of diphosphonate on glycogen content of rabbit ear cartilage cells in culture. Calcif Tissue Int 30: 163–166
Felix R, Bettex JD, Fleisch H (1981) Effect of diphosphonates on the synthesis of prostaglandins in cultured calvaria cells. Calcif Tissue Int 33: 549–552
Felix R, Guenther HL, Fleisch H (1984) The subcellular distribution of ^{14}C dichloromethylenebisphosphonate and ^{14}C 1-hydroxyethylidene-1,1-bisphosphonate in cultured calvaria cells. Calcif Tissue Int 36: 108–113
Finerman GAM, Stover SL (1981) Heterotopic ossification following hip replacement or spinal cord injury. Two clinical studies with EHDP. Metab Bone Dis Rel Res 4: 337–342
Fleisch H (1983) Bisphosphonates: mechanisms of action and clinical applications. In: Peck WA (ed) Bone and mineral research, annual 1. Excerpta Medica, Amsterdam, 319–357
Fleisch H, Bisaz S (1962) Isolation from urine of pyrophosphate, a calcification inhibitor. Am J Physiol 203: 671–675
Fleisch H, Neuman WF (1961) Mechanisms of calcification: role of collagen, polyphosphates, and phosphatase. Am J Physiol 200: 1296–1300
Fleisch H, Russell RGG (1970) Pyrophosphate and polyphosphate. In: Encyclopaedia (Int) of pharmacology and therapeutics, section 51. Pharmacology of the endocrine system and related drugs. Pergamon, Oxford, p 61
Fleisch H, Russell RGG, Straumann F (1966) Effect of pyrophosphate on hydroxyapatite and its implications in calcium homeostasis. Nature 212: 901–903
Fleisch H, Russel RGG, Francis MD (1969) Diphosphonates inhibit hydroxyapatite dissolution in vitro and bone resorption in tissue culture and in vivo. Science 165: 1262–1264
Fleisch H, Russel RGG, Bisaz S, Mühlbauer RC, Williams DA (1970) The inhibitory effect of phosphonates on the formation of calcium phosphate crystals in vitro and on aortic and kidney calcification in vivo. Eur J Clin Invest 1: 12–18
Flora L (1979) Comparative antiinflammatory and bone protective effects of two diphosphonates in adjuvant arthritis. Arthritis Rheum 4: 340–346
Flora L, Hassing GS, Parfitt AM, Villanueva AR (1980) Comparative skeletal effects of two diphosphonates in dogs. Metab Bone Dis Rel Res 2: 389–407
Fogelman I, Smith L, Mazess R, Wilson MA, Bevan JA (1986) Absorption of oral disphosphonate in normal subjects. Clin Endocrinol (Oxf.), 24: 57–62
Francis MD (1969) The inhibition of calcium hydroxyapatite crystal growth by polyphosphates. Calcif Tissue Res 3: 151–162
Francis MD, Martodam RR (1983) Chemical, biochemical, and medicinal properties of the diphosphonates. In: Hilderbrand RL (ed) The role of phosphonates in living systems. CRC, Boca Raton, Florida, p 55
Francis MD, Slough CL (1984) Acute intravenous infusion of disodium dihydrogen (1-hydroxyethylidene)diphosphonate: mechanism of toxicity. J Pharm Sci 73: 1097–1100
Francis MD, Russell RGG, Fleisch H (1969) Diphosphonates inhibit formation of calcium phosphate crystals in vitro and pathological calcification in vivo. Science 165: 1264–1266
Francis MD, Flora LF, King WF (1972) The effects of disodium ethane-1-hydroxy-1,1-diphosphonate on adjuvant induced arthritis in rats. Calcif Tissue Res 9: 109–121

Fraser D, Russell RGG, Pohler O, Robertson WG, Fleisch H (1972) The influence of disodium ethane-1-hydroxy-1,1-diphosphonate (EHDP) on the development of experimentally induced urinary stones in rats. Clin Sci 42: 197–207

Frijlink WB, Velde J te, Bijvoet OLM, Heynen G (1979) Treatment of Paget's disease with (3-amino-1-hydroxypropylidene)-1,1-bisphosphonate (A.P.D.). Lancet 1: 799

Gallagher JA, Guenther HL, Fleisch H (1982) Rapid intracellular degradation of newly synthesized collagen by bone cells. Effect of dichloromethylenebisphosphonate. Biochim Biophys Acta 719: 349–355

Garattini S (1985) Bone resorption, metastasis, and diphosphonates. Monographs of the Mario Negri Institute for pharmacological research. Raven, New York

Gasser AB, Morgan DB, Fleisch HA, Richelle LJ (1972) The influence of two diphosphonates on calcium metabolism in the rat. Clin Sci 43: 31–45

Gebauer U, Russell RGG, Touabi M, Fleisch H (1976) Effect of diphosphonates on adenosine 3′:5′ cyclic monophosphate in mouse calvaria after stimulation by parathyroid hormone in vitro. Clin Sci Mol Med 50: 473–478

Geho WB, Whiteside JA (1973) Experience with disodium etidronate in diseases of ectopic calcification. In: Frame B, Parfitt AM, Duncan H (eds) Clinical aspects of metabolic bone disease. Excerpta Medica, Amsterdam, p 506

Grabenstetter RJ, Cilley WA (1971) Polynuclear complex formation in solutions of calcium ion and ethane-1-hydroxy-1,1-diphosphonic acid. I. Complexometric an pH titrations. J Phys Chem 75: 676–682

Guenther HL, Guenther HE, Fleisch H (1979) Effects of 1-hydroxyethane-1,1-diphosphonate and dichloromethane-diphosphonate on rabbit articular chondrocytes in culture. Biochem J 184: 203–214

Guenther HL, Guenther HE, Fleisch H (1981a) The effects of 1-hydrocyethane-1,1-diphosphonate and dichloromethanediphosphonate on collagen synthesis by rabbit articular chondrocytes and rat bone cells. Biochem J 196: 293–301

Guenther HL, Guenther HE, Fleisch H (1981b) The influence of 1-hydroxyethane-1,1-diphosphonate and dichloromethanediphosphonate on lysine hydroxylation and crosslink formation in rat bone, cartilage and skin collagen. Biochem J 196: 303–310

Guilland DF, Sallis JD, Fleisch H (1974) The effect of two diphosphonates on the handling of calcium by rat kidney mitochondria in vitro. Calcif Tissue Res 15: 303–314

Guilland D, Trechsel U, Bonjour JP, Fleisch H (1975) Stimulation of calcium absorption and apparent increased intestinal, 1,25-dihydroxycholecalciferol in rats treated with low doses of ethane-1-hydroxy-1,1-diphosphonate. Clin Sci Mol Med 48: 157–160

Guncaga J, Lauffenburger R, Lentner C, Dambacher MA, Haas HG, Fleisch H, Olah AJ (1974) Diphosphonate treatment of Paget's disease of bone. A correlated metabolic, calcium kinetic and morphometric study. Horm Metab Res 6: 62–69

Gural RP (1975) Pharmacokinetics and gastrointestinal absorption behavior of etidronate. Dissertation, University of Kentucky

Hähnel H, Mühlbach R, Lindenhayn K, Schaetz P, Schmidt UJ (1973) Zum Einfluß von Diphosphonat auf die experimentelle Heparinosteopathie. Z Alternforsch 27: 289–292

Hansen NM Jr, Felix R, Bisaz S, Fleisch H (1976) Aggregation of hydroxyapatite crystals. Biochim Biophys Acta 451: 549–559

Harvey RG, Sombre ER De (1964) The Michaelis-Arbuzov and related reactions. In: Grayson M, Griffith EJ (eds) Topics in phosphorus chemistry, vol I, 3. Wiley, New York, p 57

Heaney RP, Saville PD (1976) Etidronate disodium in postmenopausal osteoporosis. Clin Pharmacol Ther 20: 593–604

Hendlin D, Stapley EO, Jackson M, Wallick H, Miller AK, Wolf FJ, Miller TW, Chaiet L, Kahan FM, Foltz EL (1969) Phosphonomycin, a new antibiotic produced by strains of streptomyces. Science 166: 122–123

Henley JW, Croxson RS, Ibbertson HK (1979) The cardiovascular system in Paget's disease of bone and the response to therapy with calcitonin and diphosphonate. Aust NZ J Med 9: 390–397

Heynen G, Delwaide P, Bijvoet OLM, Franchimont P (1982) Clinical and biological effects of low doses (3 amino-1-hydroxypropylidene)-1,1-bisphosphonate (APD) in Paget's disease of bone. Eur J Clin Invest 11: 29-35

Hilderbrand RL (1983) The effects of synthetic phosphonates on living systems. In: Hilderbrand RL (ed) The role of phosphonates in living systems. CRC, Boca Raton, p 139

Hilderbrand RL, Henderson TO (1983) Phosphonic acids in nature. In: Hilderbrand RL (ed) The role of phosphonates in living systems. CRC, Boca Raton, p 5

Hill LF, Lumb GA, Mawer EB, Stanbury SW (1973) Indirect inhibition of the biosynthesis of 1,25-dihydroxycholecalciferol in rats treated with a diphosphonate. Clin Sci 44: 335-347

Hollander W, Prusty S, Nagraj S, Kirkpatrick B, Paddock J, Colombo M (1978) Comparative effects of cetaben (PHB) and dichloromethylene diphosphonate (Cl_2MBP) on the development of atherosclerosis in the cynomoglus monkey. Atherosclerosis 31: 307-325

Horiguchi M, Kandatsu M (1959) Isolation of 2-aminoethane phosphonic acid from rumen Protozoa. Nature 184: 901-902

Jacobs TP, Siris ES, Bilezikian JP, Baquiran DC, Shane E, Canfield RE (1981) Hypercalcemia of malignancy: treatment with intravenous dichloromethylene diphosphonate. Ann Intern Med 94: 312-316

Jee WSS, Black HE, Gotcher JE (1981) Effect of dichloromethane disphosphonate on cortisol-induced bone loss in young adult rabbits. Clin Orthop Rel Res 156: 39-51

Johnson KY, Wesseler MA, Olson HM, Martodam RR, Poser JW (1982) The effects of diphosphonates on tumor-induced hypercalcemia and osteolysis in Walker carcinosarcoma 256 (W-256) of rats. In: Donath A, Courvoisier B (eds) Diphosphonates and bone. Médecine et Hygiène, Genève, p 386

Johnston CC Jr, Altman RD, Canfield RE, Finerman GAM, Taulbee JD, Ebert ML (1983) Review of fracture experience during treatment of Paget's disease of bone with etidronate disodium (EHDP). Clin Orthop 172: 186-194

Jowsey J, Holley KE, Linman JW (1970) Effect of sodium etidronate in adult cats. J Lab Clin Med 76: 126-133

Jowsey J, Riggs BL, Kelly PJ, Hoffman DL, Bordier P (1971) The treatment of osteoporosis with disodium ethane-1-hydroxy-1,1-diphosphonate. J Lab Clin Med 78: 574-584

Jung A (1982) Comparison of two parenteral diphosphonates in hypercalcemia of malignancy. Am J Med 72: 221-226

Jung A, Bisaz S, Fleisch H (1973) The binding of pyrophosphate and two diphosphonates on hydroxyapatite crystals. Calcif Tissue Res 11: 269-280

Jung A, Bornand J, Mermillod B, Edouard C, Meunier PJ (1984) Inhibition by diphosphonates of bone resorption induced by the Walker tumor of the rat. Cancer Res 44: 3007-3011

Kaplan RA, Geho WB, Pointdexter C, Haussler M, Dietz GW, Pak CYC (1977) Metabolic effects of diphosphonate in primary hyperparathyroidism. J Clin Pharmacol 17: 410-419

King WR, Francis MD, Michael WR (1971) Effect of disodium ethane-1-hydroxy-1,1-diphosphonate on bone formation. Clin Orthop 78: 251-270

Komissarenko SV, Zhuravskii NI, Karlova NP, Gulyi MF (1977) Inhibition of hypersensitivity of delayed and immediate types in guinea pigs by methylenediphosphonic acid. Bull Exp Biol Med 84: 1322-1323

Kramsch DM, Chan CT (1978) The effect of agents interfering with soft tissue calcification and cell proliferation on calcific fibrous fatty plaques in rabbits. Circ Res 42: 562-571

Labat ML, Tzehoval E, Moricard Y, Feldmann M, Milhaud G (1983) Lack of a T-cell dependent subpopulation of macrophages in (dichloromethylene) diphosphonate-treated mice. Biomed Pharmacother 37: 270-276

Labat ML, Florentin I, Davigny M, Moricard Y, Milhaud G (1984) Dichloromethylene diphosphonate (Cl_2MDP) reduces natural killer (NK) cell activity in mice. Metab Bone Dis Rel Res 5: 281-287

Lamson ML, Fox JL, Huguchi WI (1984) Calcium and 1-hydroxyethylidene-1,1-bisphosphonic acid: polynuclear complex formation in the physiological range of pH. Int J Pharmaceut 21: 143–154

Larsson A (1974) The short-term effects of high doses of ethylene-1-hydroxy-1,1-diphosphonates upon early dentin formation. Calcif Tissue Res 16: 109–127

Larsson SE (1976) The metabolic heterogeneity of glycosaminoglycans of the different zones of the epiphyseal growth plate and the effect of ethane-1-hydroxy-1,1-diphosphonate (EHDP) upon glycosaminoglycan synthesis in vivo. Calcif Tissue Res 21: 67–82

Lenehan TM, Balligand M, Nunamaker DM, Wood FE Jr (1985) Effect of EHDP on fracture healing in dogs. J Orthop Res 3: 499–507

Leonard EP, Reese WV, Mandel EJ (1979) Comparison of the effects ethane-1-hydroxy-1,1-diphosphonate and dichloromethane diphosphonate upon periodontal bone resorption in rice rats. Arch Oral Biol 24: 707–708

Levy RJ, Wolfrum J, Schoen FJ, Hawley MA, Lund SA (1985) Inhibition of calcification of bioprosthetic heart valves by local controlled-release diphosphonate. Science 228: 190–192

Liggett SJ (1973) Determination of ethane-1-hydroxy-1,1-diphosphonic acid (EHDP) in human feces and urine. Biochem Med 7: 68–77

Lockwood DR, Vogel JM, Schneider VS, Hulley SB (1975) Effect of the diphosphonate EHDP on bone mineral metabolism during prolonged bed rest. J Clin Endocrinol Metab 41: 533–541

Martodam RR, Thornton KS, Sica DA, Souza SM, Flora L, Mundy GR (1983) The effects of dichloromethylene diphosphonate on hypercalcemia and other parameters of the humoral hypercalcemia of malignancy in the rat Leydig cell tumor. Calcif Tissue Int 35: 512–519

Metzger AL, Singer FR, Bluestone R, Pearson CM (1974) Failure of disodium etidronate in calcinosis due to dermatomyositis and scleroderma. N Engl J Med 291: 1294–1296

Meunier P, Chapuy MC, Courpron P, Vignon E, Edouard C, Bernard J (1975) Effets cliniques, biologiques et histologiques de l'éthane-1-hydroxy-1,1-diphosphonate (EHDP) dans la maladie de Paget. Rev Rhum Mal Osteoartic 42: 699–705

Meunier PJ, Alexandre C, Edouard C, Mathieu L, Chapuy MC, Bressot C, Vignon E, Trechsel U (1979) Effects of disodium dichloromethylenediphosphonate on Paget's disease of bone. Lancet 2: 489–492

Meyer JL, Nancollas GH (1973) The influence of multidentate organic phosphonates on the crystal growth of hydroxyapatite. Calcif Tissue Res 13: 295–303

Meyer JL, Lee KE, Bergert JH (1977) The inhibition of calcium oxalate crystal growth by multidentate organic phosphonates. Calcif Tissue Res 23: 83–86

Michael WR, King WR, Wakim JM (1972) Metabolism of disodium ethane-1-hydroxy-1,1-diphosphonate (disodium etidronate) in the rat, rabbit, dog and monkey. Toxicol Appl Pharmacol 21: 503–515

Milhaud G, Labat ML, Moricard Y (1983) (Dichloromethylene) diphosphonate-induced impairment of T-lymphocyte function. Proc Natl Acad Sci USA 80: 4469–4473

Miller SC, Jee WSS (1979) The effect of dichloromethylenediphosphonate, a pyrophosphate analog, on bone and bone cell structure in the growing rat. Anat Rec 193: 439–462

Minaire P, Bérard E, Meunier PJ, Edouard C, Goedert G, Pilonchéry G (1981) Effects of disodium dichloromethylene diphosphonate on bone loss in paraplegic patients. J Clin Invest 68: 1086–1092

Morgan DB, Monod A, Russell RGG, Fleisch H (1973) Influence of dichloromethylene diphosphonate (Cl_2MDP) and calcitonin on bone resorption, lactate production and phosphatase and pyrophosphatase content of mouse calvaria treated with parathyroid hormone in vitro. Calcif Tissue Res 13: 287–294

Mühlbauer RC, Russell RGG, Williams DA, Fleisch H (1971) The effects of diphosphonates, polyphosphates, and calcitonin on immobilisation osteoporosis in rats. Eur J Clin Invest 1: 336–344

Mühlemann HR, Bowles D, Schatt A, Bernimoulin JP (1970) Effect of diphosphonate on human supragingival calculus. Helv Odontol Acta 14: 31-33

Nagant de Deuxchaisnes C, Rombouts-Lindemans C, Huaux JP, Devogelaer JP, Malghem J, Madlague B (1979) Roentgenologic evaluation of the action of the diphosphonate EHDP and of combined therapy (EHDP and calcitonin) in Paget's disease of bone. Mol Endocrinol 1: 405-433

Nixon GA, Buehler EV, Newmann EA (1972) Preliminary safety assessment of disodium etidronate as an additive to experimental oral hygiene products. Toxicol Appl Pharmacol 22: 661-671

Nolen GA, Buehler EV (1971) The effects of disodium etidronate on the reproductive functions and embryogeny of albino rats and New Zealand rabbits. Toxicol Appl Pharmacol 18: 548-561

Ohata M, Pak CY (1974) Preliminary study of the treatment of nephrolithiasis (calcium stones) with diphosphonate. Metabolism 23: 1167-1173

Ohya K, Yamada S, Felix R, Fleisch H (1985) Effect of bisphosphonates on prostaglandin synthesis by rat bone cells and mouse calvaria in culture. Clin Sci 69: 403-411

Pilczyk R, Sutcliffe H, Martin TJ (1972) Effects of pyrophosphate and diphosphonates on parythyroid hormone- and fluoride-stimulated adenylate cyclase activity. FEBS Lett 24: 225-228

Plasmans CMT, Kuypers W, Slooff TJJH (1978) The effect of ethane-1-hydroxy-1,1-diphosphonic acid (EHDP) on matrix induced ectopic bone formation. Clin Orthop Rel Res 132: 233-243

Plasmans CMT, Jap PHK, Kujipers W, Slooff TJJH (1980) Influence of diphosphonate on the cellular aspect of young bone tissue. Calcif Tissue Int 32: 247-256

Pollard M, Luckert PH (1985) Effects of dichloromethylene diphosphonate on the osteolytic and osteoplastic effects of rat prostate adenocarcinoma cells. JNCI 75: 949-954

Preston CJ, Yates AJP, Beneton MNC, Russell RGG, Gray RES, Smith R, Kanis JA (1986) Effective short term treatment of Paget's disease with oral etidronate. Br Med J 292: 79-80

Rabens SF, Bethune JE (1975) Disodium etidronate therapy for dystrophic cutaneous calcification. Arch Dermatol 111: 357-361

Radl J, Croese JW, Zurcher C, Enden-Vieveen MHM Van Den, Brondijk RJ, Kazil M, Haaijman JJ, Reitsma PH, Bijvoet OLM (1985) Influence of treatment with ADP-bisphosphonate on the bone lesions in the mouse 5T2 multiple myeloma. Cancer 55: 1030-1040

Recker RR, Saville PD (1973) Intestinal absorption of disodium ethane-1-hydroxy-1,1-diphosphonate (disodium etidronate) using a deconvolution technique. Toxicol Appl Pharmacol 24: 580-589

Recker RR, Hassing GS, Lau JR, Saville PD (1973) The hyperphosphatemic effect of disodium ethane-1-hydroxy-1,1-diphosphonates (EHDP™): renal handling of phosphorus and the renal response to parathyroid hormone. J Lab Clin Med 81: 258-266

Reiner M, Sautter V, Olah A, Bossi A, Largiadèr U, Fleisch H (1980) Diphosphonate treatment in myositis ossificans progressiva. In: Caniggia A (ed) Etidronate. Instituto Gentili, Pisa, p 237

Reitsma PH, Bijvoet OLM, Verlinden-Ooms H, Wee-Pals LJA van der (1980) Kinetic studies of bone and mineral metabolism during treatment with (3-amino-1-hydroxy-prophylidene)-1,1-bisphosphonate (APD) in rats. Calcif Tissue Int 32: 145-147

Reitsma PH, Teitelbaum SL, Bijvoet OLM, Kahn AJ (1982) Differential action of the bisphosphonates (3-amino-1-hydroxypropylidene)-1,1-bisphosphonate (APD) and disodium dichloromethylidene bisphosphonate (Cl_2MDP) on rat macrophage-mediated bone resorption in vitro. J Clin Invest 70: 927-933

Reynolds JJ, Minkin C, Morgan DB, Spycher D, Fleisch H (1972) The effect of two diphosphonates on the resorption of mouse calvaria in vitro. Calcif Tissue Res 10: 302-313

Reynolds JJ, Murphy H, Mühlbauer RC, Morgan DB, Fleisch H (1973) Inhibition by

diphosphonates of bone resorption in mice and comparison with grey lethal osteopetrosis. Calcif Tissue Res 12: 59–71
Robertson WG, Peacock M, Nordin BEC (1973) Inhibitors of the growth and aggregation of calcium oxalate crystals in vitro. Clin Chim Acta 43: 31–37
Rosenblum IY, Black HE, Ferrell JF (1977) The effects of various diphosphonates on a rat model of cardiac calciphylaxis. Calcif Tissue Res 23: 151–159
Russell RGG, Mühlbauer RC, Bisaz S, Williams DA, Fleisch H (1970) The influence of pyrophosphate, condensed, phosphates, phosphonates and other phosphate compounds on the dissolution of hydroxyapatite in vitro and on bone resorption induced by parathyroid hormone in tissue culture and in thyroparathyroidectomised rats. Calcif Tissue Res 6: 183–196
Russell RGG, Bisaz S, Donath A, Morgan DB, Fleisch H (1971) Inorganic pyrophosphate in plasma in normal persons and in patients with hypophosphatasia, osteogenesis imperfecta and other disorders of bone. J Clin Invest 50: 961–969
Russell RGG, Smith R, Preston C, Walton RJ, Woods CG (1974) Diphosphonates in Paget's disease. Lancet 1: 894–898
Ryzen E, Martodam RR, Troxell M, Benson A, Paterson A, Shepard K, Hicks R (1985) Intravenous etidronate in the management of malignant hypercalcemia. Arch Intern Med 145: 449–452
Schenk R, Merz WA, Mühlbauer R, Russell RGG, Fleisch H (1973) Effect of ethane-1-hydroxy-1,1-diphosphonate (EHDP) and dichloromethylene diphosphonate (Cl_2MDP) on the calcification and resorption of cartilage and bone in the tibial epiphysis and metaphysis of rats. Calcif Tissue Res 11: 196–214
Schenk R, Eggli P, Felix R, Fleisch H, Rosini S (1986) Quantitative morphometric evaluation of the inhibitory activity of new aminobisphosphonates on bone resorption in the rat. Calcif Tissue Int 38: 342–349
Schibler D, Russell RGG, Fleisch H (1968) Inhibition of pyrophosphate and polyphosphate of aortic calcification induced by vitamin D_3 in rats. Clin Sci 35: 363–372
Shane E, Baquiran DC, Bilezikian JP (1981) Effect of dichloromethylene diphosphonate on serum and urinary calcium in primary hyperparathyroidism. Ann Intern Med 95: 23–27
Shindoa H, Adamek G, Felix R, Fleisch H, Schenk R, Hagan P (1983) Structure-activity relationship of various bisphosphonates. Calcif Tissue Int 35: 87–99
Siris ES, Canfield RE, Jacobs TP, Baquiran DC (1980a) Long-term therapy of Paget's disease of bone with EHDP. Arthritis Rheum 23: 1177–1183
Siris ES, Sherman WH, Baquiran DC, Schlatterer JP, Osserman EF, Canfield RE (1980b) Effects of dichloromethylene diphosphonate on skeletal mobilization of calcium in multiple myeloma. N Engl J Med 302: 310–315
Siris ES, Hyman GA, Canfield R (1983) Effects of dichloromethylene diphosphonate in woman with breast carcinoma metastatic to the skeleton. Am J Med 74: 401–406
Sleeboom HP, Bijvoet OLM, van Oosterom AT, Gleed JH, O'Riordan JLH (1983) Comparison of intravenous (3-amino-1-hydroxypropylidene)-1,1-bisphosphonate and volume repletion in tumor-induced hypercalcemia. Lancet 2: 239–243
Slooff TJJH, Feith R, Bijvoet OLM, Nollen AJG (1974) The use of a disphosphonate in para-articular ossification after total hip replacement. A clinical study. Acta Orthop Belg 40: 820–828
Smith JD (1983) Metabolism of phosphonates. In: Hilderbrand RL (ed) The role of phosphonates in living systems. CRC, Boca Raton, p 31
Smith R, Russell RGG, Bishop M (1971) Diphosphonates and Paget's disease of bone. Lancet 1: 945–947
Spielman G, Gennarelli TA, Rogers CR (1983) Disodium etidronate: its role in preventing heterotopic ossification in severe head injury. Arch Phys Med Rehabil 64: 539–542
Steber J, Wierich P (1986) Properties of hydroxyethane disphosphonate affecting its environmental fate: degradability, sludge adsorption, mobility in soils, and bioconcentration. Chemosphere 15: 929–945

Steiner RM, Glassman L, Schwartz MW, Vanace P (1974) The radiological findings in dermatomyositis of childhood. Pediatr Radiol 111: 385–393

Stevenson PH, Stevenson JR (1986) Cytotoxic and migration inhibitory effects of bisphosphonates on macrophages. Calcif Tissue Int 38: 227–233

Storm T, Thamsborg G, Soerensen OH, Lund B (1987) The effects of etidronate therapy in postmenopausal osteoporotic women: Preliminary results. In: Christiansen C (ed) Osteoporosis 1987, International Symposium on Osteoporosis, Denmark. Norhaven A/S, Viborg

Stronski St A, Trechsel U, Fleisch H (1985) Plasma osteocalcin: lack of relation with bone resorption and effect of bisphosphonates in rats. Calcif Tissue Int 38 [Suppl]: S 39

Sturzenberger OP, Swancar JR, Reiter G (1971) Reduction of dental calculus in humans through the use of a dentifrice containing a crystal-grwoth inhibitor. J Periodontol 42: 416–419

Stutzer A, Fleisch H, Trechsel U (1987a) Long and short term effects of a single administration of bisphosphonates on retinoid induced bone resorption. J Bone Min Res 2 [Suppl] 1: 416

Stutzer A, Trechsel U, Fleisch H, Schenk R (1987b) Effect of bisphosphonates on osteoclast number and bone resorption in the rat. J Bone Min Res 2 [Suppl] 1: 266

Thiébaud D, Jaeger P, Jacquet AF, Burckhardt P (1986) A single-day treatment of tumor-induced hypercalcemia by intravenous amino-hydroxypropylidene bisphosphonate. J Bone Min Res 1: 555–562

Thomas BJ, Amstutz HC (1985) Results of the administration of diphosphonate for the prevention of heterotopic ossification after total hip arthroplasty. J Bone Joint Surg 67A: 400–403

Trechsel U, Schenk R, Bonjour JP, Russell RGG, Fleisch H (1977) Relation between bone mineralization, Ca absorption, and plasma Ca in phosphonate-treated rats. Am J Physiol 232: E298–E305

Troehler U, Bonjour JP, Fleisch H (1975) Renal secretion of diphosphonates in rats. Kidney Int 8: 6–13

Van Breukelen FJM, Bijovet OLM, Oosterom AT (1979) Inhibition of osteolytic bone lesions by (3-amino-1-hydroxypropylidene)-1,1-bisphosphonate (A.P.D.). Lancet 1: 803–805

Van Breukelen FJM, Bijvoet OLM, Frijlink WB, Sleebloom HP, Mulder H, von Oosterom AT (1982) Efficacy of amino-hydroxypropylidene bisphosphonate in hypercalcemia: observations on regulation of serum calcium. Calcif Tissue Int 34: 321–327

Van Rooijen N, van Nieuwmegen R, Kamperdijk EWA (1985) Elimination of phagocytic cells in the spleen after intravenous injection of liposome-encapsulated dichloromethylene diphosphonate. Virchows Arch [B] 49: 375–383

Walton RJ, Russell RGG, Smith R (1975) Changes in the renal and extrarenal handling of phosphate induced by disodium etidronate (EHDP) in man. J Clin Sci Mol Med 49: 45–56

Wasserman RH, Bonjour JP, Fleisch H (1973) Ileal absorption of disodium ethane-1-hydroxy-1,1-diphosphonate (EHDP) and disodium dichloromethylene diphosphonate (Cl_2MDP) in the chick. Experientia 29: 1110–1111

Wiedmer WH, Zbinden AM, Trechsel U, Fleisch H (1983) Ultrafiltrability and chromatographic properties of pyrophosphate, 1-hydroxyethylidene-1,1-bisphosphonate, and dichloromethylenebisphosphonate in aqueous buffers and in human plasma. Calcif Tissue Int 35: 397–400

Wingen F, Schmähl D (1985) Distribution of 3-amino-1-hydroxypropane-1,1-diphosphonic acid in rats and effects on rat osteosarcoma. Arzneimittelforschung 35: 1565–1571

Wink CS, Onge MSt, Parker B (1985) The effects of dichloromethylene bisphosphonate on osteoporotic femora of adult castrate male rats. Acta Anat 124: 117–121

Worms KH, Blum H (1979) Umsetzungen von 1-Aminoalkal-1,1-diphosphonsäuren mit salpetriger Säure. Z Anorg Allg Chem 457: 209–213

Worms KH, Schmidt-Dunker M (1976) Phosphonic acids and derivatives. In: Kosolapoff GM, Maier L (eds) Organic phosphorus compounds, vol 7. Wiley, New York, p 1
Yakatan GJ, Poynor WJ, Talbert RL, Floyd BF, Slough CL, Ampulski RS, Benedict JJ (1982) Clodronate kinetics and bioavailability. Clin Pharmacol Ther 31: 402–410
Yates AJP, Percival RC, Gray RES, Urwin GH, Hamdy NAT, Preston CJ, Beneton MNC, Russell RGG, Kanis JA (1985) Intravenous clodronate in the treatment and retreatment of Paget's disease of bone. Lancet 1: 1474–1477
Zernov IM, Stefani DV, Vel'tischev YE (1979) Assessment of the protective action of diphosphonate compound against damage to T-lymphocytes by antilymphocytic serum. Bull Exp Biol Med 87: 253–254

Pathophysiological Aspects and Therapeutic Approaches of Tumoral Osteolysis and Hypercalcemia

J. P. Bonjour and R. Rizzoli

Division of Clinical Pathophysiology, Department of Medicine, University Hospital, 1211 Geneva 4, Switzerland

Numerous malignant tumors can affect the skeleton and disturb the homeostasis of both calcium (Ca) and inorganic phosphate (Pi), the two main constituents of bone mineral (Rodman and Sherwood 1978; Mundy and Martin 1982). The clinical consequences of these disturbances can be dramatic on the degree of morbidity of cancer patients. Bone metastasis and osteolysis are a major source of pain, pathological fractures, and disability. Hypercalcemia is associated with nausea, vomiting, dehydration, mental disturbance, confusion, and eventually coma. The appropriate management of tumor-mediated bone osteolysis and hypercalcemia requires an appreciation of the various factors implicated in bone remodeling and in Ca homeostasis (Mundy and Roodman 1987; Bonjour et al. 1987).

Pathophysiological Aspects

The causes of malignant hypercalcemia and osteolysis have been classically enumerated in relation to both the type of tumors and the presence or absence of clinically detectable bone metastasis (Mundy and Martin 1982). They have been divided into three groups: (1) hematogenous malignancies; (2) solid tumors with bone metastasis; and (3) solid tumors without bone metastasis, also designated as humoral hypercalcemia of malignancy (HHM). This traditional classification implicated the existence of different pathophysiological mechanisms for each of these three categories of malignancies. However, as discussed below, recent evidence indicates that the same "calciotropic" factors can be produced by tumors which were until now supposed to promote bone resorption and hypercalcemia by quite different mechanisms, for instance breast cancer (group 2) and squamous cell carcinoma of the lung (group 3). Furthermore, a single type of tumoral cell can produce different factors that are able to influence either directly or indirectly bone remodeling and mineral homeostasis (Mundy and Roodman 1987; Mundy 1987). Therefore, future analysis regarding the pathogenesis of hypercalcemia and osteolysis of malignancy will have to consider: (1) the molecular nature of the causative factor(s), (2) the implicated target cell(s), and (3) the disturbed physiological function(s).

Figure 1 shows the numerous putative factors which could play a role in osteolysis and hypercalcemia of malignancy. It also shows the target organs and the main disturbed physiological functions.

Recent Results in Cancer Research, Vol. 116

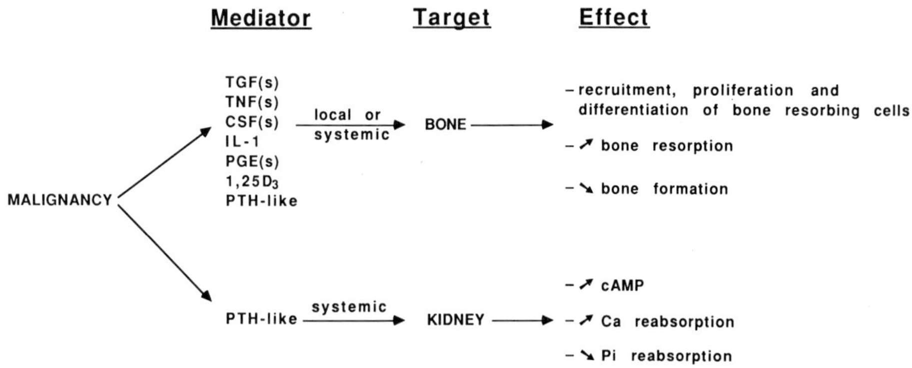

Fig. 1. Putative factors implicated in osteolysis, hypercalcemia, and hypophosphatemia of malignancy. The main target organs and physiological functions influenced by these factors are also indicated. See text for further details and abbreviations

Cytokines and Prostaglandins

Mediators such as transforming growth factors (TGFs), tumor necrosis factors (TNFs), colony-stimulating factors (CSFs), interleukin-1 (IL-1), and prostaglandins (PGEs) could be produced either directly by various types of neoplastic cells or indirectly by immune cells of the monocytic and lymphocytic lineages. These factors have been shown to stimulate osteoclastic bone resorption, at least in vitro, and some, such as TNF(s) or IL-1, could in addition exert an inhibitory effect on osteoblastic bone formation. The putative role of these various agents has been thoroughly discussed in two recent reviews (Mundy and Roodman 1987; Mundy 1987).

1,25-Dihydroxyvitamin D

The active metabolite or hormonal form of vitamin D, 1,25-dihydroxyvitamin D3 (1,25D3), has been shown to circulate in high concentration in some patients with T-cell lymphoma (Breslau et al. 1984). This finding suggests that the neoplastic T cells could have acquired the capacity of producing 1,25D3, a function which normally is essentially accomplished by specialized epithelial cells of the renal proximal tubule. Excessive circulating 1,25(OH)2D can be expected to increase the processes of both bone resorption and intestinal absorption of Ca.

Parathyroid Hormone-Like Factor(s)

Very recently considerable progress has been made regarding the chemical structure and the biological activities of tumoral factor(s) mimicking the effect of parathyroid hormone (PTH). The PTH-like or PTH-related peptide (PTHrP) factor is a molecule produced by solid tumors with and without the potentiality of metastasizing into bone. This tumoral product could increase both bone resorption and the tubular reabsorption of Ca, and decrease the tubular reabsorption of Pi. Recently, this factor (or very homologous molecules) was purified from three different types of tumors: a squamous cell carcinoma of lung (Moseley et al. 1987), a renal carcinoma (Strewler et al. 1987), and a breast carcinoma (Stewart et al. 1987). The molecule isolated from the lung tumor (Suva et al. 1987) indicates that it is composed of a single chain of 141 amino acids in which 8 of the first 13 amino acids are the same as those of PTH. Despite such an homology to the biologically active N-terminal portion of the hormone normally secreted by the parathyroid glands, the factor appears to be the product of a different gene.

At the bone level, the action of PTHrP could be similar to that of PTH, i.e., it could stimulate osteoclastic bone resorption by interacting with receptors localized in the osteoblastic cells which, in turn, would generate a factor acting directly on osteoclasts (McSheehy and Chambers 1986). As for PTH, an additional activity on the recruitment of osteoclast precursors, explaining the increase in osteoclast number, could also be invoked for PTHrP.

At the kidney level, we have recently demonstrated that conditioned medium from the same lung tumor as that from which PTHrP was isolated (Pizurki et al. 1987) was capable of both stimulating cAMP production and inhibiting the transport of Pi in cultured renal epithelial cells, in a way quite similar to synthetic PTH(1-34). The same type of response was obtained with purified PTHrP(1-141) and synthetic PTHrP(1-34) derived from this squamous cell carcinoma of the lung (Pizurki et al. 1988).

Preliminary experiments from our laboratory suggest that tumoral PTHrP(1-34) not only inhibits renal Pi reabsorption, but also stimulates the tubular reabsorption of Ca in a way similar to PTH (Rizzoli et al. 1988). Finally, like PTH, this tumoral product increases the circulating level of 1,25(OH)2D (Horiushi et al. 1987), probably by a direct action on the renal tubular cells (Ullrich Trechsel, personal communication). As illustrated in Fig. 2, it seems that squamous cell carcinoma of the lung can secrete a factor that interacts with PTH receptors and mimics in many respects the biological effects of PTH on Ca, Pi, and vitamin D metabolism at the bone and kidney levels. Other solid tumors, including kidney and breast carcinoma, could be able to secrete, at least in vitro, the same PTH-like factor.

Parathyroid hormone-related peptide could play an important role in the occurrence of hypercalcemia in solid tumors with and without bone metastasis. This peptide could contribute to the increased bone resorption which is associated with the hypercalcemia observed in most types of solid tumors (Bonjour et al. 1987). Furthermore, and probably of crucial importance, it could be the factor responsible for the increased tubular reabsorption of Ca recorded in various neoplasms during hypercalcemic episodes. It is now widely accepted that an increase in bone resorption is not the only mechanism responsible for increasing the level of blood Ca in cancer patients. An inadequate elevation of the renal tubular reabsorption of Ca plays a nonnegligible contributing role in numerous solid tumors, and even appears to be the major determinant of hypercalcemia in a subgroup of neoplasms. Note that a state of dehydration consecutive to hypercalcemia can lead to an increased renal reabsorption of both sodium and Ca. However, this mechanism

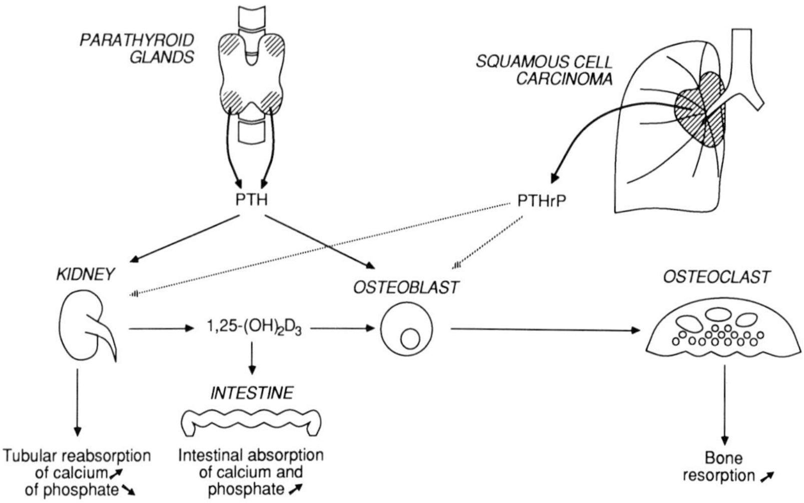

Fig. 2. Similar influence of parathyroid hormone *(PTH)* and parathyroid hormone-related peptide *(PTHrP)* on kidney and bone target cells. See text for details

cannot be implicated in many cancer patients, since a high tubular Ca reabsorption threshold is maintained despite adequate rehydration and extracellular volume expansion by profuse saline infusion (Hosking et al. 1981; Ralston et al. 1984; Bonjour et al. 1985; Percival et al. 1985). Figure 3 illustrates the relationship between plasma and urine calcium in patients with hypercalcemia of malignancy as compared with primary hyperparathyroidism.

Experimentally, a sodium-independent increase in the renal reabsorption of Ca has been clearly demonstrated in rats bearing Leydig cell tumor (LCT) (Rizzoli et al. 1986). This tumor secretes a PTH-like protein that could be PTHrP(1–141) or a close analog. In LCT-bearing rats, inhibition of tubular reabsorption of Ca by the organic thiophosphate WR-2721 (Hirschel-Scholz et al. 1985) can normalize the calcemia within hours (Hirschel-Scholz et al. 1986). In contrast, in this animal model of hypercalcemia of malignancy, bisphosphonates administered at doses completely blocking bone resorption only induce a partial reduction of the plasma level of Ca (Martodam et al. 1983). This incomplete therapeutic response is certainly related to the inability of the bisphosphonates to reverse the increased tubular reabsorption of Ca.

It is now widely accepted that increased bone resorption and increased renal tubular reabsorption of Ca can both be involved in the pathogenesis of hypercalcemia of malignancy. Recently (Bonjour et al. 1985, 1988), we have evaluated the relative importance of these two mechanisms in 33 patients with hypercalcemia of malignancy after extracellular volume expansion and after single infusion of clodronate (Cl_2MDP: 500 mg i.v. over 8 h). The fasting urine Ca/creatinine ratio was taken as an index of bone resorption (BRI). An index of the tubular reabsorption of Ca (TRCaI) was calculated from a nomogram based on the relationship between urine Ca excretion per unit of glomerular filtration rate and plasma Ca. The pathogenesis of hypercalcemia varied according to the type of neoplasm

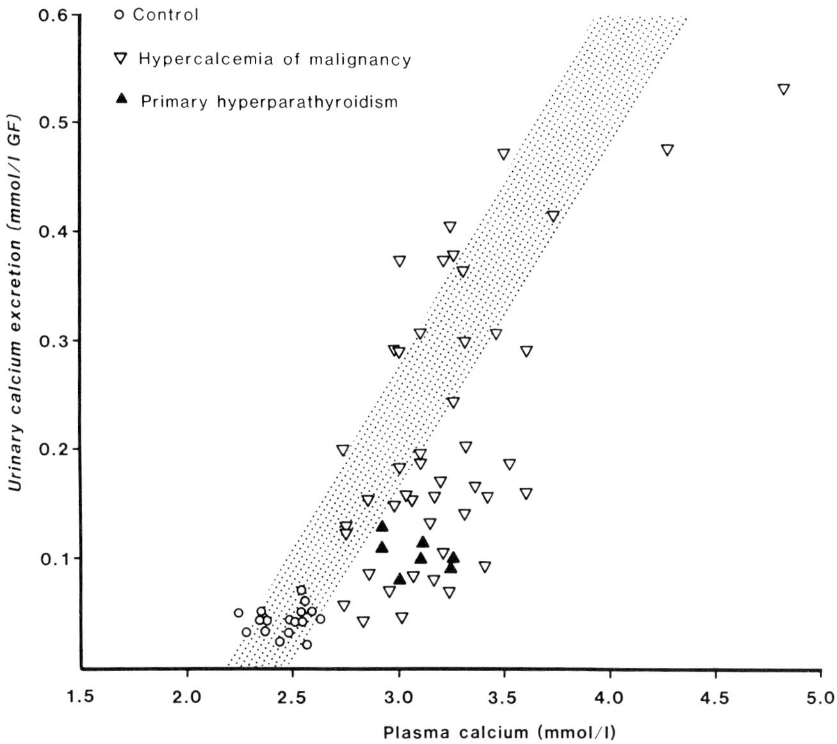

Fig. 3. Urinary excretion of Ca as a function of plasma Ca in patients with hypercalcemia of malignancy as compared with primary hyperparathyroidism. Blood and urine samples were collected in the fasted state. The *shaded area* represents the relationship obtained in normal subjects before and during the infusion of Ca. Each symbol corresponds to the mean of two determinations on consecutive days. (Adapted from Bonjour et al. 1988)

(Table 1). BRI was particularly elevated in multiple myeloma and breast tumors. TRCaI was markedly increased in squamous-cell carcinoma of the lung and in bladder, kidney, and liver neoplasms. In these tumors TRCaI reached levels observed in primary hyperparathyroidism. TRCaI was normal in most cases of multiple myeloma. Breast tumors appeared to be heterogeneous with respect to TRCaI, ranging from normal to very high values. This latter finding is quite interesting in relation to the recent isolation from a breast carcinoma of a PTH-like protein (Stewart et al. 1987). In our studies, mean (±SEM) plasma Ca fell from 3.29 ± 0.07 to 2.69 ± 0.05 mmol/liter 3 days after Cl_2MDP ($n=33$, $P<0.001$), a response similar to that obtained with repeated daily i.v. injections of 500–1000 mg Cl_2MDP (Jung 1982). The fall in plasma Ca in response to Cl_2MDP was usually most marked in cancer patients with elevated BRI and normal TRCaI. It was often quite modest in patients with high TRCaI and slightly elevated BRI. Thus, a stimulation of bone resorption is not the only mechanism of the maintenance of hypercalcemia of malignancy. In some tumors characterized by a poor response to bisphosphonate administration, at least when given in a single infu-

Table 1. Mean indices of bone resorption *(BRI)* and tubular reabsorption of Ca *(TRCaI)* in several types of neoplasms with hypercalcemia

	BRI (UCa/Ucreat.) (mmol/mmol)	TRCaI (mmol/liter GFR)	Plasma Ca (mmol/liter)
Normal range	0.16–0.50	2.36–2.86	2.25–2.62
Myeloma	1.30*	2.64	3.21
Lymphoma	2.99*	2.51	3.02
Breast carcinoma	2.65*	2.99*	3.35
Kidney carcinoma	0.98	3.20*	3.30
Lung carcinoma (squamous cells)	1.13	2.98*	2.98
Primary hyperpara-thyroidism	0.92	3.07*	3.07

For each type of neoplasm, the most elevated index as compared with normal range is marked by an asterisk: it probably corresponds to the prevailing component(s) responsible for the elevation of plasma Ca. In breast carcinoma both bone resorption and tubular reabsorption of Ca appear to play a contributing role. The corresponding individual values for the various neoplasms are presented in Fig. 4. (Data adapted from Bonjour et al. 1988)

sion, a marked enhancement in the tubular reabsorption of Ca appears to be the prevailing mechanism for hypercalcemia (Bonjour et al. 1988). Table 1 shows the mean values for BRI, TRCaI, and plasma Ca found in several types of malignancies and, for comparison, in primary hyperparathyroidism. The individual values are presented in Fig. 4. In virtually all patients BRI was above the normal range. However, in 63% TRCaI was also abnormally elevated.

Therapeutic Approaches

In hypercalcemia of malignancy, when the osteolytic or calciotropic tumoral product(s) cannot be suppressed by anticancer therapy, treatment should be mainly aimed at correcting the disturbed Ca flux(es). As mentioned above, in most cases a stimulation in net bone resorption is involved. Theoretically, two rational approaches could be envisaged: stimulation of Ca deposition into bone and/or inhibition of bone resorption. Today there is no available pharmacological agent able to increase bone formation rapidly and thereby to sequestrate the excess Ca present in the extracellular pool.

Agents Affecting Bone Resorption

Several agents are available for inhibiting bone resorption. Calcitonin can be effective in some cases, particularly when it is given with glucocorticoids (Binstock and Mundy 1980). However, its effect is of short duration (Ljunghall et al. 1987). In contrast, treatment with bisphosphonate (Fleisch 1983) is of benefit in the majority of patients with hypercalcemia of malignancy. As compared with calci-

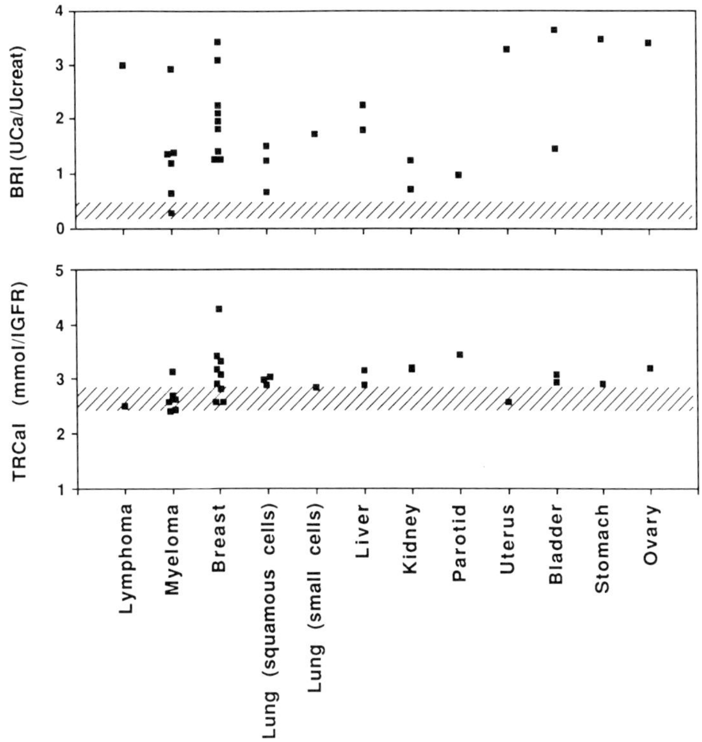

Fig. 4. Individual values of bone resorption *(BRI)* and tubular reabsorption of Ca *(TRCaI)* indices in several types of neoplasms with hypercalcemia. Each symbol corresponds to the index calculated in individual patients after rehydration, but before antiosteolytic therapy with clodronate. (Data adapted from Bonjour et al. 1988)

tonin, bisphosphonates are capable of maintaining a normal plasma level of Ca over a prolonged period (Ljunghall et al. 1987). Most reports on bisphosphonates published so far concern three compounds: 1-hydroxyethane-1-1 bisphosphonic acid (HEBP), dichloromethylenebisphosphonic acid (Cl_2MBP), and 3-amino-1-hydroxypropane-1, 1-bisphosphonic acid (APD). They have been given either orally or intravenously (Bonjour et al. 1987). Until now all bisphosphonates evaluated in hypercalcemia of malignancy have been shown to be effective, at least when administered intravenously every day for 7–10 days. However, a single infusion of Cl_2MBP or APD delivered over a few hours seems to be as effective, at least in the short term, as daily injections repeated during 1 week. This observation does not mean that the maintenance of normocalcemia is not dependent upon the amount of bisphosphonate accumulated in the bone. However, the exact relationship between the bisphosphonate skeletal content and the duration of bone resorption inhibition is not known. As mentioned above a poor response to bisphosphonate therapy can be occasionally observed in adequately rehydrated patients. It could be mostly due to their inability to reduce the renal reabsorption of Ca in patients with PTHrP-secreting tumors. Nevertheless a resistance at the bone level can also occasionally be observed.

Recently, gallium nitrate has been shown to be effective in hypercalcemia of malignancy (Warrel et al. 1986). A preliminary report indicates that this compound could inhibit bone resorption in vitro (Bockman et al. 1986). In our laboratory we have recently observed that gallium nitrate inhibits retinoid-induced bone resorption in vivo (unpublished observation). This newcomer to the antiosteolytic arsenal deserves to be further evaluated and compared with the bisphosphonates of the current (Cl_2MBP, HEBP, APD) and new generation (4-amino-1-hydroxybutylidene-1, 1-bisphosphonic acid, 6-amino-1-hydroxyhexylidene-1, 1-bisphosphonic acid, azacycloheptylidene-2, 2-bisphosphonic acid, (chloro-4 phenyl) thiomethylene bisphosphonic acid, 2(2-pyridyl)ethylidene-1, 1-bisphosphonic acid) (Fleisch 1987).

Agents Affecting Tubular Ca Reabsorption

As mentioned above, in hypercalcemia of malignancy, an increased tubular reabsorption of Ca could be due to two different mechanisms: (a) enhanced reabsorption of sodium resulting from dehydration and extracellular volume contraction and (b) secretion by the tumoral cells of a PTH-like molecule acting selectively on the transport of Ca without affecting that of sodium. It is obvious that a rational therapeutic approach should consider which of these pathophysiological mechanisms is responsible for the anomaly in the renal handling of Ca. In the former case, restoration and maintenance of a normal hydration state by intravenous saline infusion is the treatment of choice. In the second case, a selective normalization of the tubular reabsorption of Ca should be achieved. However, such a therapeutic goal is still difficult to reach with the pharmacological tools available today. Until now the combination of profuse saline infusion with diuretics such as furosemide has been used. This approach is not only of dubious efficacy for reducing the tubular reabsorption of Ca, but it can also have dangerous consequences on electrolyte and fluid balance. Calcitonin, alone (Hosking and Gilson 1984) or combined with a glucocorticoid (Ralston et al. 1985), might be able to interfere with the renal hypercalcemic component. Such a treatment seems to be a much safer approach than the use of excessive saline infusions combined with powerful natriuretic agents. Nevertheless, what is badly needed in these cases displaying a hyperparathyroidism-like syndrome is a specific inhibitor of the tubular reabsorption of Ca which does not affect the renal transport of sodium. With the recent molecular identification of the tumoral PTHrP, there is some hope that analogs with antagonist property can be synthesized and be active in vivo. In the meantime the only experimental agent which appears to have the property of reducing the tubular reabsorption of Ca is the organic thiophosphate WR-2721 (Hirschel-Scholz et al. 1985, 1986). This radioprotective agent could be useful not only in the medical management of hyperparathyroidism (Hirschel-Scholz and Bonjour 1987) but also in the treatment of tumor-mediated hypercalcemia with markedly enhanced renal reabsorption of Ca. Figure 5 summarizes the main therapeutic tools that have been shown so far to influence the fluxes of Ca at the intestinal, skeletal, and renal levels in preclinical and clinical investigations.

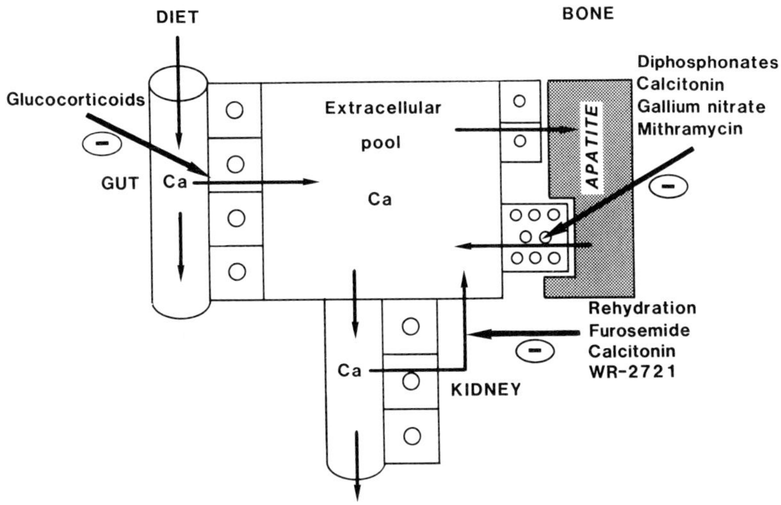

Fig. 5. Main therapeutic tools for influencing calcium fluxes in osteolysis and hypercalcemia of malignancy. Gallium nitrate and WR-2721 (*S*-, 2-(3-aminopropylamino)-, ethylphosphorothioic acid) are investigational drugs that deserve to be further evaluated in hypercalcemia of malignancy

Summary

Malignant tumors can affect the integrity of the skeletal tissue and the homeostasis of the two main components of bone mineral, calcium (Ca) and inorganic phosphate (Pi). Various tumoral cell products can increase bone resorption by influencing the number of osteoclasts and/or their activity. These tumoral products could act either directly on bone cells of the osteoblastic or osteoclastic lineages, or indirectly by influencing cells secreting osteotropic factors, such as interleukin-1, tumor necrosis factors, transforming growth factors, and colony-stimulating factor. Among the classical calciotropic hormones, 1,25-dihydroxyvitamin D3 could be implicated in lymphoma. In hypercalcemia of malignancy, an increase in bone resorption is observed in most patients. However, in many cases an increased tubular reabsorption of Ca has been documented as well. This phenomenon when present after adequate rehydration is probably due to the secretion by the tumoral cells of a parathyroid hormone-related peptide (PTHrP). This factor has been recently identified as a protein containing 141 amino acids. This protein or some very close analogs have been shown to be secreted by lung, kidney and also breast carcinoma. Besides increasing bone resorption and stimulating tubular reabsorption of Ca, PTHrP also selectively decreases the tubular reabsorption of Pi, an action that may explain the hypophosphatemia observed in some types of neoplasm.

Therapeutically, administration of antiresorbing agents such as clodronate or other bisphosphonates can normalize the increased osteolysis and, if present, the associated elevation in the plasma level of Ca in most cancer patients. However in some cases, wherein the prevailing hypercalcemic mechanism is due to an enhancement in the tubular reabsorption of Ca, other therapeutic means should be associated with the antiosteolytic bisphosphonate therapy.

Acknowledgments. The work from our research group discussed in this article was supported by the Swiss National Foundation (grant 3.954.0.85), the Elsie and Carlos de Reuter Foundation, and the League against Cancer from Geneva. The authors wish to thank Mrs. Marie-Christine Brandt for preparing the manuscript.

Part of the data presented in Table 1, Fig. 3, and Fig. 4 are reprinted from *Bone*, Vol. 9 No. 3, pp. 123–130, 1988: Bonjour J.-P., Philippe J., Bisetti A., Rizzoli R., Jung A., Rosini S., and Kanis J., "Bone and renal components in hypercalcemia of malignancy and responses to a single infusion of clodronate", Copyright 1988, Pergamon Journals Ltd.

References

Binstock ML, Mundy GR (1980) Effect of calcitonin and glucocorticoids in combination on the hypercalcemia of malignancy. Ann Intern Med 93: 269–272

Bockman RS, Boskey A, Alcock N, Bullough P, Warrell R (1986) Gallium nitrate inhibits bone resorption, increases bone calcium content but is not cytotoxic to bone cells (abstract). J Bone Min Res 1: 65

Bonjour JP, Philippe J, Guelpa G, Bisetti A, Rizzoli R, Jung A, Rosini S (1985) Bone and renal components in hypercalcemia of malignancy (HM) evaluated in relation with the therapeutical response to one single infusion of clodronate. Calcif Tissue Int 38 [Suppl]: S32

Bonjour JP, Rizzoli R, Hirschel-Scholz S, Caverzasio J (1987) Management of hypercalcemia in relation to pathophysiology. Bone 8 [Suppl 1]: S29–S33

Bonjour JP, Philippe J, Guelpa G, Bisetti A, Rizzoli R, Jung A, Rosini S, Kanis JA (1988) Bone and renal components in hypercalcemia of malignancy and responses to a single infusion of clodronate. Bone 9: 123–130

Breslau NA, McGuire JL, Zerwekh JE, Frenkel EP, Pak CYC (1984) Hypercalcemia associated with increased serum calcitriol levels in three patients with lymphoma. Ann Intern Med 100: 1–7

Fleisch H (1983) Bisphosphonates: mechanisms of action and clinical applications. In: Peck WA (ed) Bone and mineral research/1. Excerpta Medica, Amsterdam, pp 319–357

Fleisch H (1987) Bisphosphonates – history and experimental basis. Bone 8 [Suppl 1]: S23–S28

Hirschel-Scholz S, Bonjour JP (1987) Radioprotective agent WR-2721 opens new perspective in treatment of hyperparathyroidism and hypercalcemia. Trend Pharmacol Sci 8: 246–247

Hirschel-Scholz S, Caverzasio J, Bonjour JP (1985) Inhibition of parathyroid hormone (PTH) secretion and PTH-independent diminution of tubular Ca reabsorption by WR-2721, a unique hypocalcemic agent. J Clin Invest 76: 1851–1856

Hirschel-Scholz S, Caverzasio J, Rizzoli R, Bonjour JP (1986) Normalization of hypercalcemia associated with a decrease in renal calcium reabsorption in Leydig cell tumor-bearing rats treated with WR-2721. J Clin Invest 78: 319–322

Horiuchi N, Caulfield MP, Fisher JE, Goldman ME, McKee RL, Reagan JE, Levey JJ, Nutt RF, Rodan SB, Schofield TL, Clemens TL, Rosenblatt M (1987) Similarity of synthetic peptide from human tumor to parathyroid hormone in vivo and in vitro. Science 238: 1566–1570

Hosking DJ, Gilson D (1984) Comparison of the renal and skeletal actions of calcitonin in the treatment of severe hypercalcemia of malignancy. Q J Med 211: 359–368

Hosking DJ, Cowley A, Bucknall CA (1981) Rehydration in the treatment of severe hypercalcaemia. Q J Med 200: 473–481

Jung A (1982) Comparison of two parenteral diphosphonates in hypercalcemia of malignancy. Am J Med 72: 221-227
Ljunghall S, Rastad J, Akerstrom G (1987) Comparative effects of calcitonin and clodronate in hypercalcaemia. Bone 8 [Suppl 1]: S79-S83
Martodam RR, Thornton KS, Sica DA, D'Souza SM, Flora L, Mundy GR (1983) The effects of dichloromethylene diphosphonate on hypercalcemia and other parameters of the humoral hypercalcemia of malignancy in the rat Leydig cell tumor. Calcif Tissue Int 35: 512-519
McSheehy PMJ, Chambers TJ (1986) Osteoblastic cells mediate osteoclastic responsiveness to parathyroid hormone. Endocrinology 118: 824-828
Moseley JM, Kubota M, Diefenbach-Jagger H, Wettenhall REH, Kemp BE, Suva LJ, Rodda CP, Ebeling PR, Hudson PJ, Zajac JD, Martin TJ (1987) Parathyroid hormone-related protein purified from a human lung cancer cell line. Proc Natl Acad Sci USA 84: 5048-5052
Mundy GR (1987) Bone resorption and turnover in health and disease. Bone 8 [Suppl 1]: S9-S16
Mundy GR, Martin TJ (1982) The hypercalcemia of malignancy. Pathogenesis and management. Metabolism 31: 1247-1277
Mundy GR, Roodman GD (1987) Osteoclast ontogeny and function. In: Peck WA (ed) Bone and mineral research/5. Elsevier, Amsterdam, pp 209-279
Percival RC, Yates AJP, Gray RES, Galloway J, Rogers K, Neal FE, Kanis JA (1985) Mechanism of malignant hypercalcaemia in carcinoma of the breast. Br Med J 291: 776-779
Pizurki L, Rizzoli R, Caverzasio J, Bonjour JP (1987) Specific inhibition by parathyroid hormone-like factor(s) produced by human lung squamous-cell carcinoma of sodium-dependent phosphate transport in cultured renal epithelium. J Bone Min Res 2 [Suppl 1]: 393 (Abstract)
Pizurki L, Rizzoli R, Moseley J, Martin TJ, Caverzasio J, Bonjour JP (1988) Effect of synthetic tumoral parathyroid hormone related peptide on cAMP production and sodium-dependent phosphate transport in cultured renal cells epithelia (abstract). Calcif Tissue Int 42 [Suppl 2]: A46
Ralston SH, Dryburgh FJ, Cowan RA, Gardner MD, Jenkins AS, Boyle IT (1985) Comparison of aminohydroxypropylidene diphosphonate, mithramycin, and corticosteroids/calcitonin in treatment of cancer-associated hypercalcaemia. Lancet 2: 907-910
Rizzoli R, Caverzasio J, Fleisch H, Bonjour JP (1986) Parathyroid hormone-like changes in renal calcium and phosphate reabsorption induced by Leydig cell tumor in thyroparathyroidectomized rats. Endocrinology 119: 1004-1009
Rizzoli R, Caverzasio J, Moseley J, Martin TJ, Vadas L, Bonjour JP (1988) Synthetic tumoral parathyroid hormone related peptide (PTHrP(1-34)) stimulates the renal tubular reabsorption of calcium (TRCa) (abstract). J Bone Min Res 3 [Suppl 1]: no. 13
Rodman JS, Sherwood LM (1978) Disorders of mineral metabolism in malignancy. In: Avioli LV, Krane SM (eds) Metabolism bone diseases. Academic, New York, pp 577-631
Stewart AF, Burtis WJ, Wu T, Goumas D, Broadus AE (1987) Two forms of parathyroid hormone-like adenylate cyclase-stimulating protein derived from tumors associated with humoral hypercalcemia of malignancy. J Bone Min Res 2: 587-593
Strewler GJ, Stern PH, Jacobs JW, Eveloff J, Klein RF, Leung SC, Rosenblatt M, Nissenson RA (1987) Parathyroid hormone-like protein from human renal carcinoma cells. Structural and functional homology with parathyroid hormone. J Clin Invest 80: 1803-1807
Suva LJ, Winslow GA, Wettenhall REH, Hammonds RG, Moseley JM, Diefenbach-Jagger H, Rodda CP, Kemp BE, Rodriguez H, Chen EY, Hudson PJ, Martin TJ, Wood WI (1987) A parathyroid hormone-related protein implicated in malignant hypercalcemia: cloning and expression. Science 237: 893-896
Warrell RP Jr, Skelos A, Alcock NW, Bockman RS (1986) Gallium nitrate for acute treatment of cancer-related hypercalcemia: clinicopharmacological and dose response analysis. Cancer Res 46: 4208-4212

*Use of Clodronate and Calcitonin in Hypercalcemia Due to Malignancy**

S. Ljunghall

Department of Internal Medicine, University Hospital, 75185 Uppsala, Sweden

Introduction

Malignant tumours frequently cause hypercalcemia through both renal and skeletal mechanisms (Bonjour et al. 1988). Tumor-associated bone resorption can be localized, generalized, or both and is characterized clinically by destructive osteolytic bone metastases. It has become clear that tumors may produce several factors which stimulate osteoclastic bone resorption, leading to hypercalcemia, even in the absence of metastases to bone (Stewart et al. 1980; Mundy and Martin 1982; Mundy 1985; Burtis et al. 1988). Other mechanisms also contribute to the maintenance of elevated calcium levels. Hypercalcemia itself has complex effects on renal function and, apart from the impairment of glomerular filtration, enhances renal tubular calcium reabsorption (Hosking et al. 1981; Percival et al. 1985; Bonjour et al. 1988).

Both calcitonin and clodronate are agents which affect osteoclastic bone resorption and they can therefore be used in the treatment of patients with hypercalcemia associated with malignancy (Ljunghall et al. 1987). Treatment with calcitonin has been practiced for several years, whereas clodronate is not as widely available for general use. There are no direct comparative studies between these two agents.

This paper describes the effects of clodronate and calcitonin from a perspective dominated by the practical clinical needs, i.e., to reduce symptomatic hypercalcemia, regardless of its cause, and to maintain normal or near-normal serum calcium values over a prolonged time with a minimum of side effects. A basis for this comparison is drawn from an extensive review of calcitonin therapy given by Hosking and Bijvoet (1982) to which some recent studies have been added (Adachi et al. 1986; Kimura et al. 1986; Warrell et al. 1988). This is compared to data from patients treated with clodronate (Chapuy et al. 1980; Douglas et al. 1980; Jacobs et al. 1981; Shane et al. 1982; Jung 1982; Jung et al. 1983; Siris et al. 1983; Paterson et al. 1983; Percival et al. 1985; Conte et al. 1985; Witte et al. 1987; Rastad et al. 1987; Canfield et al. 1987; Urwin et al. 1987; Scharla et al. 1987; Lind et al. 1987).

* This work was supported by the Swedish Medical Research Council.

Recent Results in Cancer Research, Vol. 116

Acute Hypocalcemic Effects

During treatment with calcitonin there is great variation in the degree and completeness of response. A considerable proportion of this variation can be explained by the severity of hypercalcemia. The review on calcitonin therapy (Hosking and Bijvoet 1982) clearly demonstrated that the decrement in serum calcium attained was most pronounced in those patients with the highest pretreatment serum calcium concentrations. This is not surprising since hypercalcemia is likely to be related in part to the prevailing rate of bone resorption.

There is also a close correlation between the degree of hypercalcemia and the reduction of serum calcium achieved by clodronate. With both intravenous and oral administration of clodronate there is a more marked decrease of serum calcium than with calcitonin. Although doses have been adjusted individually, most patients appeared to respond to a dose of 1600–3200 mg of clodronate daily given orally or a dose of 300–400 mg infused intravenously over at least 3 h.

In the case of calcitonin, it has been shown that the mean reduction of hypercalcemia (the excess above 2.5 mmol/l) was about 60%, independent of the absolute pretreatment values. In other words, treatment with calcitonin did not generally result in a normalization of serum calcium levels, and the response achieved depended on the degree of the pretreatment hypercalcemia (Fig. 1).

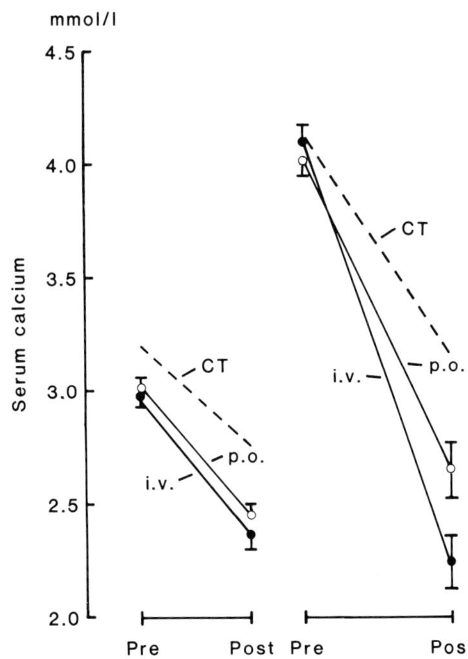

Fig. 1. Reduction of serum calcium in patients treated with oral *(p.o.)* or intravenous *(i.v.)* clodronate. Patients were subdivided according to their pretreatment serum calcium values into those whose hypercalcemia was moderate (≦3.5 mmol/l; $n=73$; *left panel*) or marked (>3.50 mmol/l; $n=42$; *right panel*). The *broken lines* show the effects of calcitonin in the corresponding groups of patients as reviewed by Hosking and Bijvoet (1982)

It further appeared that the rate of administration of the hormone was clearly of importance. Whereas a single injection of calcitonin only produced a mean reduction of hypercalcemia of around 40%, continuous infusion reduced excess calcemia by almost 80%, and many patients then achieved normal or nearly normal values. The superiority of the continuous infusion of calcitonin (in saline) over repeated injections may result in part from volume repletion and the decreased proximal calcium reabsorption induced by the saline vehicle.

The pooled data from the patients treated with clodronate, on the other hand, demonstrated that it was possible to achieve normal serum calcium values in most patients, regardless of the degree of pretreatment hypercalcemia. Oral administration of clodronate was clearly more effective than calcitonin, and intravenous administration of the bisphosphonate produced an even more pronounced response (see Fig. 1). Thus, the mean percentage reduction of hypercalcemia was close to 100% even in those patients with the more marked hypercalcemia.

Duration of Effect with Continued Administration

The effects of calcitonin on bone resorption appear to be transient both in vitro (Wener et al. 1972) and in vivo (Binstock and Mundy 1980). This has been called the "escape" phenomenon and may be due to down-regulation of receptors on bone cells occuring in the continuous presence of calcitonin. When calcitonin has been used as a single agent, the duration of response has been limited to a few days (Binstock and Mundy 1980; Hosking 1980). This "escape" phenomenon can be prevented in vitro by the addition of glucocorticoids (Raisz et al. 1972). The combination of glucocorticoids and calcitonin in one study (Binstock and Mundy 1980) made it possible to maintain the lower serum calcium concentrations over a 4-day study period. Longer term studies of calcitonin as therapy for malignancy-associated hypercalcemia have not been reported.

In contrast, there are several reports describing a sustained hypocalcemic action of clodronate. Among more than 50 published cases (Douglas et al. 1980; Paterson et al. 1983; Percival et al. 1985; Rastad et al. 1987; Lind et al. 1987) which have been followed for more than 2 weeks, a hypocalcemic response was sustained. The life expectancy of patients with hypercalcemia due to solid tumours is short, as the marked elevation of serum calcium is often a sign of advanced disease. Nevertheless, it was possible, in some patients, to maintain normal serum calcium levels over several months using orally administered clodronate. Concomitant treatment may occasionally have contributed to the prolonged response, but in several instances attempts to reduce or withdraw clodronate treatment resulted in prompt return of hypercalcemia, indicating that the underlying disturbance remained. In terminal stages hypercalcemia can recur despite ongoing treatment with clodronate; it is then presumably mainly due to enhanced renal conservation of calcium.

Side Effects

Some patients receiving calcitonin or clodronate complain of mild to moderate gastrointestinal symptoms, such as nausea and intestinal upset. Calcitonin injections or infusions may also produce temporary flushing. In the clinical management of patients with severe symptomatic hypercalcemia associated with malignancy such side effects are not easily discernible and considering the seriousness of the underlying disorder generally acceptable to the patient. In these respects, calcitonin and clodronate appear similar.

Some bisphosphonates [ethane hydroxy bisphosphonate (disodium etidronate)] may induce osteomalacia, since they impair mineralization of normal bone when given in high doses over long periods. Clodronate does not seem to have any effect on the mineralization of newly formed osteoid tissue in doses that inhibit bone resorption (Minaire et al. 1981).

Many patients with severe hypercalcemia also have impaired renal function. The nephrotoxicity of drugs given to patients with progressive renal impairment is difficult to assess but there is no evidence to suggest that calcitonin, by itself, has any adverse effect on renal function. Large intravenous bolus injections of bisphosphonates can induce structural renal abnormalities in dogs (Hintze and D'Amato 1982). When smaller doses (up to 300 mg daily) were given by intravenous infusion over some hours, no deleterious effects of clodronate on renal function were observed, even when given to patients with significantly impaired renal function (Kanis et al. 1983). In most of the patients described in detail in the literature there was either an improvement in or unchanged renal function when hypercalcemia was reversed by clodronate. In a few patients (Bounameaux et al. 1983) who have been treated with intravenous clodronate for very severe hypercalcemia, however, an impairment of already disturbed renal function has been observed. In rare instances it is not possible to exclude entirely a causal relationship with clodronate. On the other hand, in several other reported patients with progressive renal failure there was a reversal of the elevated serum creatinine levels during continuous therapy with clodronate, occurring in parallel with normalization of serum calcium levels. There is apparently no documented case of sustained renal insufficiency attributable to clodronate.

In conclusion, from the clinical point of view clodronate is a very useful adjunct to the other available therapy for malignancy-associated hypercalcemia. It has an acute hypocalcemic effect in most patients and normocalcemia can generally be maintained during long-term therapy using oral administration.

Summary

Increased bone resorption and increased renal tubular reabsorption of calcium are involved in the pathogenesis of hypercalcemia of malignancy. Clodronate and calcitonin inhibit bone resorption and have been used as therapy for malignancy-associated hypercalcemia. Both drugs induce significant reductions of serum calcium but the decrease is greater with clodronate, particularly when given intravenously. While the response to calcitonin generally is of short duration, clodronate can maintain normal serum calcium values over several weeks when oral administered.

Thus, from the clinical point of view clodronate is a very useful adjunct to the available therapy.

References

Adachi I, Kimura S, Yamaguchi K, Suzuki M, Abe K (1986) Synthetic salmon calcitonin as an antihypercalcemic agent for hypercalcemia in malignancy (in Japanese; English abstract). Gan To Kagaku Ryoho 13: 2637-2644

Binstock ML, Mundy GR (1980) Effect of calcitonin and glucocorticoids in combination on the hypercalcemia of malignancy. Ann Int Med 93: 269-272

Bonjour JP, Philippe J, Guelpa G, Bisetti A, Rizzoli R, Jung A, Rosini S, Kanis J (1988) Bone and renal components in hypercalcemia of malignancy and responses to a single infusion of clodronate. Bone 9: 123-130

Bounameaux HM, Schifferli J, Montani J-P, Jung A, Chatelanat F (1983) Renal failure associated with intravenous diphosphonates. Lancet i: 471

Burtis WJ, Wu TL, Insogna KL, Stewart AF (1988) Humoral hypercalcemia of malignancy. Ann Int Med 108: 454-457

Canfield RE, Siris ES, Jacobs TP (1987) Dichloromethylene diphosphonate action in hematologic and other malignancies. Bone 8 [Suppl 1]: S57-S62

Chapuy MC, Meunier PJ, Alexandre CM, Vignon EP (1980) Effects of disodium dichloromethylene diphosphonate on hypercalcemia produced by bone metastases. J Clin Invest 65: 1243-1247

Conte N, Di Virgilio R, Roiter I, Caberlotto L (1985) Hypercalcemia in malignancies: treatment with dichloromethylene diphosphonate (Cl_2MDP). Tumori 71: 51-54

Douglas DL, Russell RGG, Preston CJ, Prenton MA, Duckworth T, Kanis JA, Preston FE, Woodhead JS (1980) Effect of dichloromethylene diphosphonate in Paget's disease of bone and in hypercalcaemia due to primary hyperparathyroidism or malignant disease. Lancet i: 1043-1047

Hintze KL, D'Amato RA (1980) Comparative toxicology of two diphosphonates. Toxicologist 2: 192

Hosking DJ (1980) Treatment of severe hypercalcaemia with calcitonin. Metab Bone Dis Rel Res 2: 207-212

Hosking DJ, Bijvoet OLM (1982) Therapeutic uses of calcitonin. In: Parsons JA (ed) Endocrinology of calcium metabolism. Raven, New York, pp 485-535

Hosking DJ, Cowley A, Bucknall CA (1981) Rehydration in the treatment of severe hypercalcaemia. Q J Med 50: 473-481

Jacobs TP, Siris ES, Bilezikian JP, Baquiran DC, Shane E, Canfield RE (1981) Hypercalcemia of malignancy: treatment with intravenous dichloromethylene diphosphonate. Ann Intern Med 94: 312-316

Jung A (1982) Comparison of two parenteral diphosphonates in hypercalcemia of malignancy. Am J Med 72: 221-262

Jung A, Chantraine A, Donath A, van Ouwenaller C, Turnill D, Mermillod B, Kitler ME (1983) Use of dichloromethylene diphosphonate in metastatic bone disease. N Engl J Med 308: 1499-1501

Kanis JA, Preston CJ, Yates AJP, Percival RC, Mundy KI, Russell RGG (1988) Effects of intravenous diphosponates on renal function. Lancet i: 1328

Kimura S, Sato Y, Matsubara H, Adachi I, Yamaguchi K, Suzuki M, Suemasu K, Abe K (1986) A retrospective evaluation of the medical treatment of malignancy-associated hypercalcemia. Jpn J Cancer Res 77: 85-91

Lind L, Wengle B, Ljunghall S (1987) Treatment with clodronate in patients with hypercalcemia secondary to malignancy. Ups J Med Sci 92: 259-263

Ljunghall S, Rastad J, Åkerström G (1987) Comparative effects of clodronate and calcitonin in hypercalcemia. Bone 8 [Suppl 1]: S79–S84

Minaire P, Berard E, Meunier PJ, Edouard C, Goedert G, Pilonchery G (1981) Effects of disodium dichloromethylene diphosphonate on bone loss in paraplegic patients. J Clin Invest 68: 1086–1092

Mundy GR (1985) Pathogenesis of hypercalcaemia of malignancy. Clinical Endocrinology 23: 705–714

Mundy GR, Martin TJ (1982) The hypercalcemia of malignancy: pathogenesis and management. Metabolism 31: 1247–1277

Paterson AD, Kanis JA, Cameron EC, Douglas DL, Beard DJ, Preston FE, Russell RGG (1983) The use of dichloromethylene diphosphonate for the management of hypercalcaemia in multiple myeloma. Br J Haematol 54: 121–132

Percival RC, Paterson AD, Yates AJP, Beard DJ, Douglas DL, Neal FE, Russell RGG, Kanis JA (1985) Treatment of malignant hypercalcaemia with clodronate. Br J Cancer 51: 665–669

Raisz LG, Trummel CL, Wener JA, Simmons H (1972) Effect of glucocorticoids on bone resorption in tissue culture. Endocrinology 90: 961–967

Rastad J, Benson L, Johansson H, Knuutila M, Pettersson B, Wallfelt C, Åkerström G, Ljunghall S (1987) Clodronate treatment in patients with malignancy-associated hypercalcemia. Acta Med Scand 221: 489–494

Scharla SH, Minne HW, Sattar P, Mande U, Blind E, Schmidt-Gayk H, Wüster C, Ho T, Ziegler R (1987) Therapie der Tumorhypercalcaemie mit Clodronat. Einfluß auf Parathormon und Calcitriol. Dtsch Med Wochenschr 112: 1121–1125

Shane E, Jacobs TP, Siris ES, Steinberg SF, Stoddart K, Canfield RE, Bilezikian JP (1982) Therapy of hypercalcemia due to parathyroid carcinoma with intravenous dichloromethylene diphosphonate. Am J Med 72: 939–944

Siris ES, Hyman GA, Canfield RE (1983) Effects of dichloromethylene diphosphonate in women with breast carcinoma metastatic to the skeleton. Am J Med 74: 401–406

Stewart AF (1983) Therapy of malignancy-associated hypercalcemia. Am J Med 74: 475–480

Stewart AF, Horst R, Deftos LJ, Cadman EC, Lang R, Broadus AE (1980) Biochemical evaluation of patients with cancer associated with hypercalcemia: evidence for humoral and nonhumoral groups. N Engl J Med 303: 1377–1383

Urwin GH, Yates AJ, Gray RE, Hamdy NA, McCloskey EV, Preston FE, Greaves FE, Neil FE, Kanis JA (1987) Treatment of the hypercalcaemia of malignancy with intravenous clodronate. Bone 8 [Suppl 1]: S79–S84

Warrell RP Jr, Israel R, Frisone M, Snyder T, Gaynor JJ, Bockman RS (1988) Gallium nitrate for acute treatment of cancer-related hypecalcemia. A randomized double-blind comparison to calcitonin. Ann Intern Med 108: 669–674

Wener JA, Gorton SJ, Raisz LG (1972) Escape from inhibition of resorption in cultures of fetal bone treated with calcitonin and parathyroid hormone. Endocrinology 90: 752–759

Witte RS, Koeller J, Davis TE, Benson AB, Durie BG, Lipton A, Stock JL, Citrin DL, Jacobs TP (1987) Clodronate, a randomized study in the treatment of cancer-related hypercalcemia. Arch Intern Med 147: 937–939

Treatment of Tumor Hypercalcemia with Clodronate

R. Ziegler and S. H. Scharla

Abteilung für Innere Medizin I, Medizinische Universitätsklinik,
Bergheimer Straße 58, 6900 Heidelberg, FRG

Introduction

The association of hypercalcemia and malignant disease has been observed especially in patients with multiple myeloma and carcinomas of the lung, kidney, breast, prostate, and ovary (Myers 1960). As therapeutic regimens in the treatment of malignant disorders have been improved in recent years, resulting in prolonged survival of patients, humoral hypercalcemia of malignancy has become a more frequent and often serious complication of tumor disease, which requires additional treatment. Plasma calcium concentration can be lowered by isotonic sodium chloride infusions, calcitonin, prednisone, mithramycin, and oral phosphorus. However, congestive heart failure, escape phenomenon, or severe side effects can limit the duration of their application. Therefore, bisphosphonates such as etidronate or clodronate, which are known to inhibit osteoclast activity (Delaissé et al. 1985; Schenk et al. 1973), are under current clinical investigation to prove their effectivenes in hypercalcemia of malignancy. Etidronate, which is already used in the treatment of Paget's disease (Holz et al. 1983) and heterotopic ossification (Garland et al. 1983), has been demonstrated to be beneficial also in tumor hypercalcemia by several authors (Kanis et al. 1987; Ringenberg and Ritch 1987). However, besides the desired inhibition of osteolysis, etidronate also causes impairment of mineralization (Schenk et al. 1973), which may cause fractures (Canfield et al. 1977). By contrast, clodronate does not induce a skeletal mineralization defect up to an oral dose of 2.4 g daily (Delmas et al. 1982), but seems to be very effective in tumor hypercalcemia (Cohen et al. 1981; Jacobs et al. 1981; Percival et al. 1985; Siris et al. 1980). In our study we evaluated the effect of intravenous and oral clodronate administration including the reaction of the calcium-regulating hormones parathyroid hormone (PTH) and 1.25-dihydroxycholecalciferol ($1{,}25(OH)_2D_3$).

Patients and Methods

In an open controlled study we treated 34 patients with tumor hypercalcemia of different origin: mammary cancer ($n=19$), bronchus carcinoma ($n=4$), hypernephroma ($n=2$), multiple myeloma ($n=2$), uterus carcinoma ($n=2$), pancreatic carcinoma ($n=1$), melanoma ($n=1$), epithelial carcinoma of the mouth ($n=1$),

Recent Results in Cancer Research, Vol. 116

epithelial carcinoma of the vulva ($n=1$), and liver carcinoma ($n=1$). The ages of the patients were between 31 and 72 years (mean age, 56 years). Informed consent was given by all patients. Hypercalcemia persisted at least 3 days before clodronate treatment started. Five patients had received calcitonin without a lasting calcium-lowering effect. Seven patients received glucocorticoids within a protocol of polychemotherapy without increasing doses. Tumor treatment schedules like radiation or chemotherapy were continued during our efforts to lower plasma calcium.

The initial dosage of clodronate was 300 mg/day intravenously, added to 500 ml saline and infused over at least 2 h. After achieving normocalcemia (2–6 days after the start of treatment in most cases) clodronate administration was continued orally using 400–3200 mg/day depending on plasma calcium. Mostly, treatment lasted for 3 weeks, but in some cases up to 6 months.

Control parameters were plasma and urinary calcium, phosphorus, and creatinine (measured by automated routine methods). Furthermore, in 21 patients PTH (1–84) (measured by a two-site immunoradiometric assay (Blind et al. 1987) and $1{,}25(OH)_2D_3$ (quantitated by radioimmunoassay after sample purification with HPLC (Scharla et al. 1984)) were controlled. For correlation with PTH or $1{,}25(OH)_2D_3$ the plasma calcium values were corrected for protein concentration. For comparison of pre- and post-treatment values the *t*-test for paired samples was used. Side effects of clodronate were monitored by determination of routine blood parameters and physical examination as usual.

Results and Discussion

Intravenous clodronate decreased serum calcium concentration from 3.30 ± 0.41 mmol/liter to 2.44 ± 0.33 mmol/liter within 1 week. Figure 1 shows the pattern of plasma calcium concentrations during treatment. Only 6/34 patients still had calcium levels above the normal range, 4 of them reaching normocalcemia a few days later. During oral clodronate administration there was a renewed slight rise of plasma calcium (2.72 ± 0.45 mmol/liter after 3 weeks of treatment). Six patients could be observed for periods of more than 20 weeks. Two of them remained normocalcemic even after withdrawal of clodronate therapy, three received clodronate and had normal plasma calcium levels, and one patient exhibited hypercalcemia despite clodronate administration. The reincrease of calcium in most cases was an indicator of deterioration. Fifteen out of 34 patients died within the observation time because of progressive tumor disease and concomitant cachexia.

The decrease in plasma calcium was followed by a fall in calciuria (Fig. 2). This was accompanied by normalization of previously elevated plasma creatinine values documenting the improvement of renal function (Fig. 3).

Parathyroid hormone (1–84) concentration was low or subnormal in all hypercalcemic tumor patients (Fig. 4, right). Lowering of plasma calcium led to an increase in PTH (1–84); in some patients PTH (1–84) reached somewhat elevated levels. This is in accordance with the observation by some authors of secondary hyperparathyroidism in patients with bisphosphonate therapy (Delmas et al. 1982; Harris et al. 1982; Papapoulos et al. 1986).

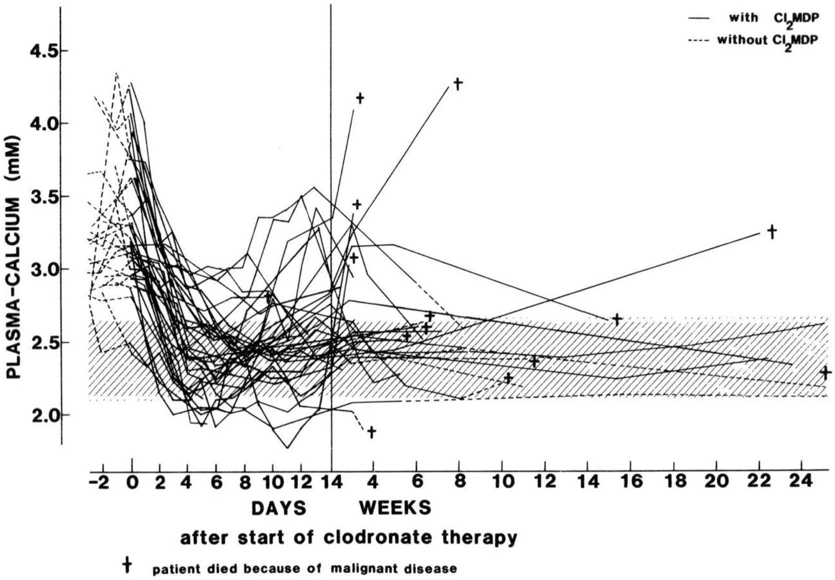

Fig. 1. Plasma calcium of 34 patients with tumor-induced hypercalcemia. Treatment started at day 0 with daily intravenous infusions of 300 mg clodronate. After achievement of normal calcium values the therapy was continued by oral clodronate administration at 400–3200 mg/day. The *shaded* area indicates the normal range for plasma calcium

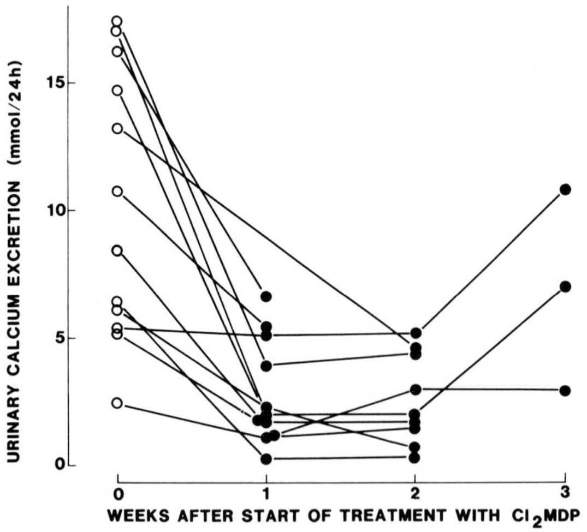

Fig. 2. Urinary excretion of calcium in 12 unselected patients with hypercalcemia of malignancy. Urine samples were collected during a 24-h period. The patients received a low-calcium diet and their tumor treatment. The range of urinary calcium excretion for normal persons on a regular diet is 2.5–5.0 mmol/24 h. Clodronate *(Cl_2MDP)* treatment resulted in a marked decrease of urinary calcium excretion in our patients

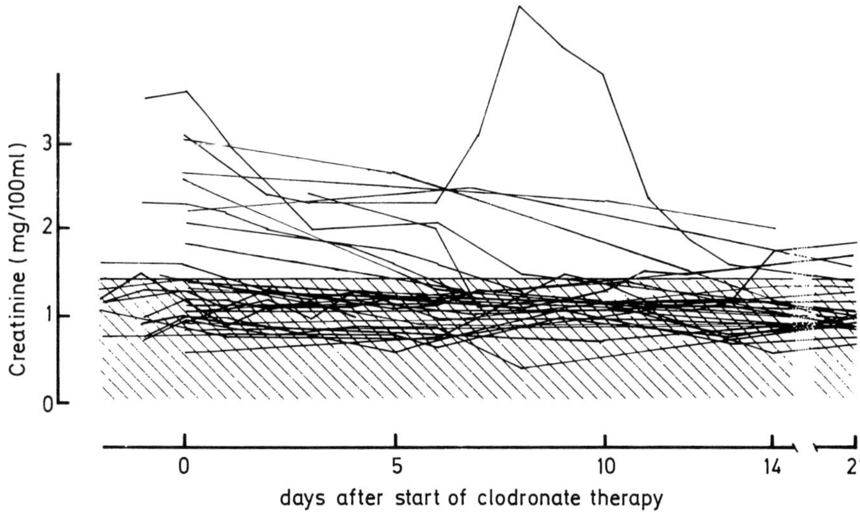

Fig. 3. Plasma creatinine in patients with hypercalcemia of malignancy. Those patients with elevated creatinine values prior to clodronate treatment exhibit improvement of renal function during clodronate administration. The marked increase in creatinine in one patient was related to a bacterial sepsis due to venous catheterization and was reversible by antibiotic therapy

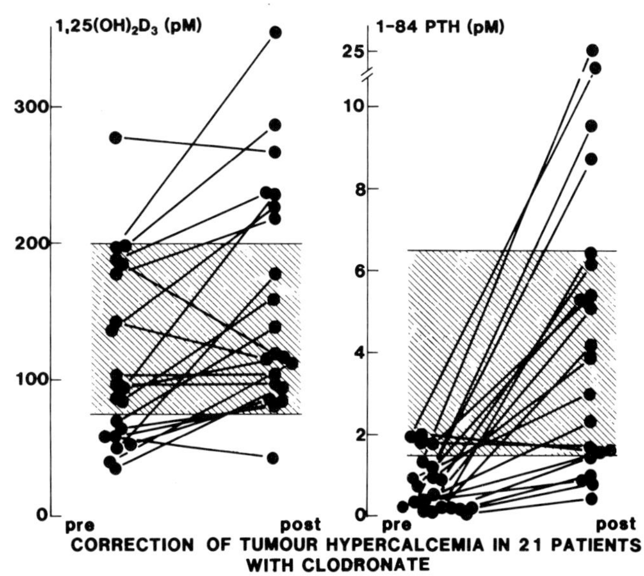

Fig. 4. 1,25-Dihydroxyvitamin D_3 *(1,25-$(OH)_2D_3$)* and intact PTH 1-84 in 21 patients with hypercalcemia of malignancy measured before start of clodronate treatment and after correction of hypercalcemia. Lowering of plasma calcium by clodronate treatment resulted in an increase of both 1,25$(OH)_2D_3$ and PTH 1-84. It should be noted that in some hypercalcemic patients 1,25$(OH)_2D_3$ was not suppressed prior to treatment despite low PTH values. *Shaded* areas indicate the respective normal ranges for 1,25$(OH)_2D_3$ and PTH 1-84

Before the start of clodronate therapy $1{,}25(OH)_2D_3$ was in the lower normal range or subnormal in 15/21 patients. In 6/21 patients $1{,}25(OH)_2D_3$ was in the upper normal range or elevated despite hypercalcemia (Fig. 4, left). There is a negative exponential correlation ($P \leq 0.02$) between plasma calcium and PTH (1-84) (Fig. 5) and a negative linear correlation ($P \leq 0.05$) between calcium and $1{,}25(OH)_2D_3$ (Fig. 6). However, there is no significant correlation between PTH (1-84) and $1{,}25(OH)_2D_3$ (Fig. 7). These data document that the relationship between plasma calcium and its regulating hormones PTH and $1{,}25(OH)_2D_3$ is not disturbed during tumor hypercalcemia and treatment with clodronate. However, stimulation of renal 1α-hydroxylase by tumor products leading to elevation of plasma $1{,}25(OH)_2D_3$ has to be considered in some patients (see above), which would explain the missing correlation between PTH and $1{,}25(OH)_2D_3$. Increased concentrations of $1{,}25(OH)_2D_3$ have been reported from patients with renal cell carcinoma-associated hypercalcemia (Yamamoto et al. 1987). In our collective there were only two patients with hypernephroma, one of them having a high plasma $1{,}25(OH)_2D_3$ concentration.

During treatment with clodronate we observed no significant changes in the function of vital organs. Clodronate did not cause significant changes of hemoglobin, erythrocytes, leukocytes, sodium, chloride, phosphorus, total protein, and aminotransferases. Only three patients had gastrointestinal complaints upon oral administration of clodronate, leading to discontinuation of treatment in one case.

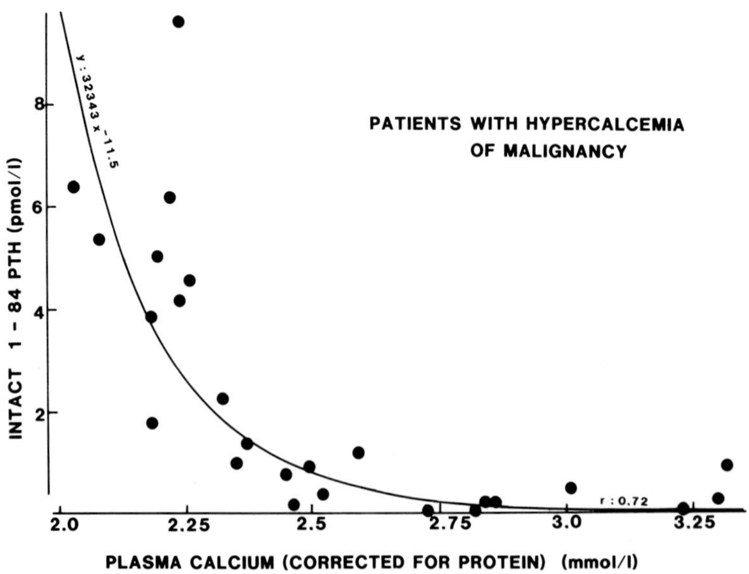

Fig. 5. Nonlinear correlation of corrected plasma calcium values and PTH concentrations in patients with hypercalcemia of malignancy ($P < 0.01$). The data were obtained both before and during clodronate treatment

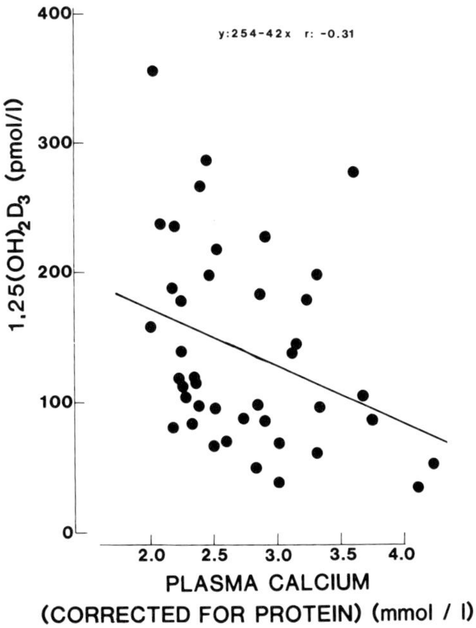

Fig. 6. Linear correlation of corrected plasma calcium values and concentrations of 1,25(OH)$_2$D$_3$ in 21 patients with tumor hypercalcemia ($P < 0.05$). The data were obtained both before and during clodronate treatment

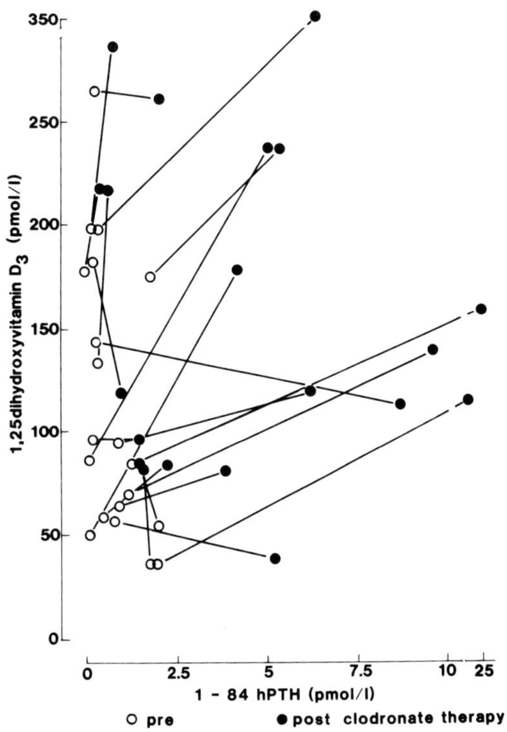

Fig. 7. Lack of a significant correlation between 1,25(OH)$_2$D$_3$ and PTH in patients with tumor hypercalcemia. *Open circles* represent data obtained prior to clodronate administration and *closed circles* the corresponding data after normalization of plasma calcium with clodronate

Conclusions

Clodronate proved to be a very efficient drug for lowering serum calcium in patients with tumor hypercalcemia. Normocalcemia contributed to clinical improvement of the patients – however, the fate depending on tumor progression was not altered. The drug was well tolerated, and there were no serious side effects.

Summary

In an open, controlled study 34 patients with tumor hypercalcemia of different origin were treated with clodronate. The initial dosage was 300 mg intravenously daily. After achieving normocalcemia, treatment was continued orally using 400–3200 mg/day depending on serum calcium concentration. Most patients showed normocalcemia within 1 week of treatment – only few of them needed a longer time. Fifteen of 34 patients died within the observation time of up to 24 weeks, some being normocalcemic. However, a reincrease in plasma calcium during treatment was an indicator of deterioration. Measurements of plasma parathyroid hormone (PTH) using an intact molecule radioimmunometric assay showed depressed levels before clodronate treatment started, but PTH rose after achieving normal and especially low normal calcium levels. Starting 1,25-dihydroxycholecalciferol [$1,25(OH)_2D_3$] values were decreased or in the lower normal range in the majority of patients, but in 6/21 patients plasma $1,25(OH)_2D_3$ was in the upper normal range or elevated despite hypercalcemia. After lowering plasma calcium the $1,25(OH)_2D_3$ levels increased. However, there was no significant correlation between PTH and $1,25(OH)_2D_3$. Therefore we assume that in some patients additional stimulation of renal 1α-hydroxylase by tumor products is present.

References

Blind E, Schmidt-Gayk H, Armbruster FP, Stadler A (1987) Measurement of intact human Parathyrin by an extracting two-site immunoradiometric assay. Clin Chem 33: 1376–1381

Canfield R, Rosner W, Skinner J, McWhorter J, Resnick L, Feldman F, Kammerman S, Ryan K, Kunigonis M, Bohne W (1977) Diphosphonate therapy of Paget's disease of bone. J Clin Endocrinol Metab 44: 96–106

Cohen AL, Koeller J, Davis TE, Citrin DL (1981) Iv dichloromethylene diphosphonate in cancer – associated hypercalcemia: a phase I–II evaluation. Cancer Treat Rep 65: 651–653

Delaissé J-M, Eeckhout Y, Vaes G (1985) Bisphopshonates and bone resorption: effects on collagenase and lysosomal enzyme excretion. Life Sci 37: 2291–2296

Delmas PD, Chapuy MC, Vignon E, Charhon S, Briancon D, Alexandre C, Edouard C, Meunier PJ (1982) Long term effects of dichloromethylene diphosphonate in Paget's disease of bone. J Clin Endocrinol Metab 54: 837–844

Garland DE, Alday B, Venos KG, Vogt JC (1983) Diphosphonate treatment for heterotopic ossification in spinal cord injury patients. Clin Orthop Rel Res 176: 197–200

Harris ST, Neer RM, Segre GV, Petkan AJ, Tully III GL, Daly M, Potts JT Jr (1982) Secondary hyperparathyroidism associated with dichloromethane diphosphonate treatment of Paget's disease. J Clin Endocrinol Metab 55: 1100–1107

Holz G, Delling G, Ziegler R (1983) Etidronsäure-Therapie bei Morbus Paget des Skelettes. Dtsch Med Wochenschr 108: 1954–1958

Jacobs TP, Siris ES, Bilezikian JP, Baquiran DC, Shane E, Canfield RE (1981) Hypercalcemia of malignancy. Treatment with intravenous dichloromethylene diphosphonate. Ann Intern Med 94: 312–316

Kanis JA, Urwin GH, Gray RES, Beneton MNC, McCloskey EV, Handy NAT, Murray SA (1987) Effects of intravenous etidronate disodium on skeletal and calcium metabolism. Am J Med 82 [Suppl 2A]: 55–70

Myers WPL (1960) Hypercalcemia in neoplastic disease. Arch Surg 80: 308–318

Papapoulos SE, Harinck HIJ, Bijvoet OLM, Gleed JH, Fraher LJ, O'Riordan JLH (1986) Effects of decreasing serum calcium on circulating parathyroid hormone and vitamin D metabolites in nomocalcaemic and hypercalcaemic patients treated with APD. Bone Mineral 1: 69–78

Percival RC, Paterson AD, Yates P, Beard DJ, Douglas DL, Neal FE, Russell RGG, Kanis JA (1985) Treatment of malignant hypercalcaemia with clodronate. Br J Cancer 51: 665–669

Ringenberg QS, Ritch PS (1987) Efficacy of oral administration of etidronate disodium in maintaining normal serum calcium levels in previously hypercalcemic cancer patients. Clin Ther 9: 319–325

Scharla S, Schmidt-Gayk H, Reichel H, Mayer E (1984) A sensitive and simplified radioimmunoassay for 1,25-dihydroxyvitamin D_3. Clin Chim Acta 142: 325–338

Schenk R, Merz WA, Mühlbauer R, Russell RGG, Fleisch H (1973) Effect of ethane-1-hydroxy-1, 1-diphosponate (EHDP) and dichloromethylene diphosphonate (Cl_2MDP) on the calcification and resorption of cartilage and bone in the tibial epiphysis and metaphysis of rats. Calcif Tissue Res 11: 196–214

Siris ES, Sherman WH, Baquiran DC, Schlatterer JP, Ossermann EF, Canfield RF (1980) Effects of dichloromethylene diphosphonate on skeletal mobilization of calcium in multiple myeloma. N Engl J Med 302: 310

Yamamoto I, Kitamura A, Aoki J, Kawamura J, Dokoh S, Morita R, Torizuka K (1987) Circulating 1,25-dihydroxyvitamin D concentrations in patients with renal cell carcinoma – associated hypercalcemia are rarely suppressed. J clin Endocrinol Metab 64: 175–179

Treatment of Tumor-Induced Osteolysis by APD

P. Burckhardt, D. Thiébaud, L. Perey, and V. von Fliedner

Departement für Innere Medizin, Universitätsklinik CHUV, 1011 Lausanne, Switzerland

Introduction

Hypercalcemia is the cause of severe clinical symptoms, such as nausea and vomiting, dehydration, renal failure, disorientation, and coma, and it can be lethal. It is primarily caused by malignant diseases (Fisken et al. 1980). Hypercalcemia of malignancy, also called "hypercalcemia of cancer," "malignant hypercalcemia," or "tumor-induced hypercalcemia," is one of the most common metabolic complications of cancer (Mundy et al. 1984), and its cumulative incidence has been estimated at around 10% (Blomqvist 1986). It occurs in a great variety of cancers, in some cases independently of the presence of detectable bone metastases, especially in squamous cell carcinoma of the lung ("humoral hypercalcemia of cancer") (Mundy et al. 1984). It is primarily due to increased bone resorption, and to a lesser degree in some tumors to increased tubular reabsorption of calcium, especially in squamous cell cancer. It is potentiated by dehydration.

The increase of bone resorption is caused by a stimulation of osteoclasts, due either to metastatic tumor cells at the endosteal surfaces, producing prostaglandines or other factors, or to circulating factors such as cytokines, interleukin 1, growth factors, osteoclast-activating factor, tumor necrosis factors, and various other growth factors and parathyroid hormone (PTH) - like peptides, the latter also stimulating tubular calcium reabsorption (Mundy 1985; Mundy et al. 1984).

Because of the clinical relevance of severe hypercalcemia, treatment is indicated. Rehydration is essential, but usually insufficient. Therapeutic drugs acting on osteoclastic bone resorption are of major use. The use of drugs with another pharmacological impact is declining. Among known osteoclast inhibitors, mithtamycin and calcitonin are not optimal, due to toxicity and short action, respectively (Sleebom and Bijvoet 1985). With the introduction of bisphosphonates, it became evident that the action of these compounds was more pronounced and more prolonged, tolerance being excellent (Van Breukelen et al. 1979). Bisphosphonates normalized plasma calcium in most patients and were finally also used for the prevention and amelioration of pain and fracture rate due to bone metastases. Various compounds were developed, such as EHDP and Cl_2MDP, the former being less potent (Adami et al. 1982). Aminobisphosphonates, including APD (3-amino-1-hydroxypropylidene-1, 1-bisphosphonate), appeared to be particularly effective (Body 1984) in inhibiting bone resorption, with no adverse effect on bone formation. This paper describes the authors' experience with this drug, and compares it with that of others.

Recent Results in Cancer Research, Vol. 116

General Experiences with APD

The literature includes a total of about 350 patients with malignant hypercalcemia treated with APD (Table 1). Initial doses were between 15 and 30 mg/day, diluted mostly in 500 ml normal saline and infused over 2-6 h, for 3-11 days. Subsequently, the doses varied between 15 and 60 mg, and the drug was given for a few days. Finally, it was given in a single infusion over 2-24 h (Coleman and Rubens 1987). Thirty to 60 mg given in one or two infusions normalized plasma calcium in most cases within 3-7 days, depending on the initial plasma calcium level. This effect was independent of the tumor type of of the presence of bone metastases (Body et al. 1986; Yates et al. 1987; Thiébaud et al. 1986; Portman et al. 1983). Plasma calcium always decreased with an almost constant slope, from the 2nd day on, and remained elevated if the initial plasma calcium was extremely elevated and/or the dose relatively small, e.g., 15 mg. A dose-efficacy relationship was demonstrated by two studies using short treatments with various doses (Thiébaud et al. 1988; Body et al. 1987). Normalization of plasma calcium, including transient slight and asymptomatic hypocalcemia, was achieved in over 90% of the cases with either 15 mg/day over 4-6 days or 60 mg in a single 24-h infusion. Maximal efficacy was achieved with a total dose of 90 mg given in one slow infusion or over 2-3 days. As a single infusion, 90 mg appears to be indicated only for very severe hypercalcemia of about 4.0 mmol/liter or more.

Considering all the published studies, there was a relationship between the total dose administered and the success rate (Table 2, Fig. 1). The success of treatment is related to both the initial plasma calcium level and the dose selected. Severe hypercalcemia requires higher doses for normalization than moderate hypercal-

Table 1. Treatment of malignant hypercalcemia by APD i.v.

References	Year of publication	Number of patients	Dose (mg/day)	Number of days
Sleeboom et al.	1983	19	15	3-10
Portmann et al.	1983	14	±25	4-11
Ralston et al.	1985	13	15	±6
Body et al.	1986	24	15	4-9
Ralston et al.	1986	8	15	±6
Thiébaud et al.	1986b	10	30	6
Stevens	1987	2	15	4+5
Body et al.	1987	18	0.1-180	3
Yates et al.	1987	11	15, 25	2-6
		16	15-30	1
Harinck et al.	1987	132	15	3-10
Coleman and Rubens	1987	22	15	1 or more
Thiébaud et al.	1986a	20	30, 60	1
Cantwell and Harris	1987	16	30	1
Jodrell et al.	1987	1	30	1
Thiébaud et al.	1987	+32	30, 45, 60, 90	1
Total	1983-1987:	358 patients		

Table 2. Success rate (percent age of patients with normalized plasma calcium) at various dose regimens. (Data from the literature[a])

Dose/day (mg/day)	Number of days	Total dose (mg)	Success rate	%	Reference
±2.9	2.4 (1-3)	7.0	4/9	44	(Coleman and Rubens 1987; Body et al. 1987)[b]
15	2.1 (1-3)	31.5	22/31	71	(Coleman and Rubens 1987; Yates et al. 1987; Body et al. 1987)
15	5.0 (4-6)	75	3/4	75	(Yates et al. 1987; Stevens 1987)
15	±6.5	97.5	57/58	98	(Body et al. 1986; Sleebom et al. 1983; Papapoulos et al. 1986)
15	ca. 4.5 (3-10)	ca. 67.5	119/132	90	(Harnick et al. 1987)
25	1.2 (1-2)	30	6/18	33	(Yates et al. 1987)
25	±5.6	140	14/14	100	(Portmann et al. 1983)[c]
30	1	30	25/32	78	(Thiébaud et al. 1988; Cantwell and Harris 1987; Yates et al. 1987; Jordell et al. 1987)
30	6.2 (4-10)	186	12/12	100	(Thiébaud et al. 1986; Sleebom et al. 1983)
45	3	135	3/3	100	(Body et al. 1987)
45	1	45	10/14	71	(Thiébaud et al. 1988)
60	1	60	13/14	93	(Thiébaud et al. 1988)
90	3	180	3/3	100	(Body et al. 1987)
90	1	90	12/12	100	(Thiébaud et al. 1988)

[a] Where dose and duration of treatment was available for individual patients.
[b] Dose indicated in milligrams per kilogram; assumed total dose for body wt. of 60 kg.
[c] Duration of treatment until normal plasma calcium on 2 days which was reached between days 3 and 4. Not longer than 10 days.

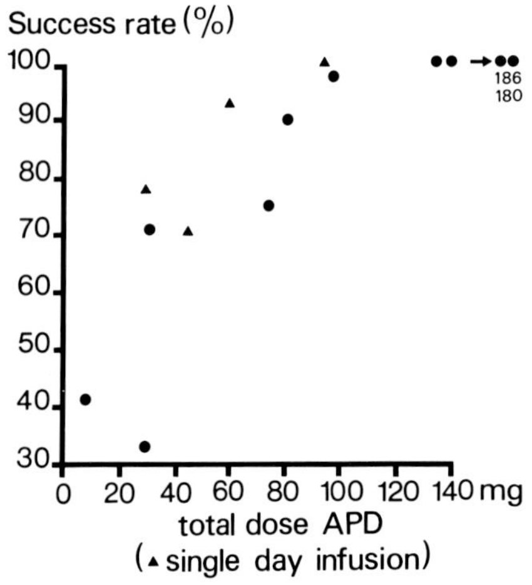

Fig. 1. Correlation between the total dose of APD adminstered (daily dose × no. of days) and the percentage of patients whose plasma calcium was normalized (transient slight hypocalcemia included), from a total of 358 patients taken from the literature (see Table 1)

cemia. The drop of calcium is almost constant and clearly does not depend on the dose or the duration of the treatment.

Urinary hydroxyproline, a specific breakdown product from collagen, is a marker of bone resorption. It decreases when bone resorption is inhibited, but not to normal values because of the increased collagen turnover within the tumor and its soft tissue metastases. This was observed in all patients. Urinary calcium excretion dropped to low levels. Urinary and plasma phosphate decreased too. This reflects a positive balance for both phosphate and calcium, and probably a positive bone balance. Plasma creatinine was lowered in most patients, in addition to the initial effect of rehydration, as the consequence of the normalization of plasma calcium. Therefore, APD can be given when plasma creatinine is elevated, at least up to twice the normal limit.

Symptoms due to hypercalcemia, such as nausea, vomiting, polydypsia, confusion, drowsiness, and coma, disappear in most patients treated. Slight asymptomatic hypocalcemia remained for one or more days in about one-fourth of the patients. Transient increase of body temperature of about 1 °C on the 2nd day for 1 or 2 days also remained unnoticed by the 18% of patients where it was measured. The transient decrease in the lymphocyte count by about 25% in 1 out of 10 patients also had no harmful consequences. No interactions were observed with other antihypocalcemic or antitumoral drugs.

Compard with other hypocalcemic agents (e.g., calcitonin, furosemide, mithramycin), APD has a prolonged effect, due to a high affinity to bone. The duration of normocalcemia and the recurrence rate of hypercalcemia did not depend on the type of malignant disease. On average, normocalcemia lasted for 3 weeks. After treatment with small doses, e.g., 30 mg in a single infusion, urinary hydroxyproline (and to a lesser extent urinary calcium) reincreased after 2 weeks, but plasma clacium still remained normal. This reincrease was not observed after a high dose 60–90 mg. In the case of recurrence, the treatment could be repeated. Only in end-stage cancer did efficacy decline.

Personal Experiences with APD

APD has been used in the authors' institution for several years. In an initial study on 14 hypercalcemic patients with various cancers (Portman et al. 1983), APD was given at a fixed daily dose of 25 mg until plasma calcium was normal for two consecutive days. All patients normalized their plasma calcium on average after 5.6 days. The daily decrease in calcium was almost identical in all patients. Therefore, the duration of treatment (and by that the total dose) depended exclusively on the initial level of plasma calcium. Total dose varied between 100 and 275 mg.

In a second study, the duration and the dose were fixed, and the drug was given either per os or i.v. to ten patients each (Thiébaud et al. 1986b). Thirty milligrams i.v. for 6 days was equipotent to 1200 mg per os for 6 days. Both groups normalized their plasma calcium at exactly the same time. This showed superiority of the intravenous treatment: equal efficacy by avoiding the gastrointestinal side effects, known from the long-term use of APD in Paget's disease (Harinck et al. 1987a). As bisphosphonates accumulate easily in the skeleton and cannot be metabolized, and as no recurrence of increased bone resorption has been observed for over 1 year in patients who were treated for mild Paget's disease by a short course of APD (Thiébaud et al. 1987), the effect of a single infusion was tested in malignant hypercalcemia.

Altogether, 68 patients (33 women and 35 men) with tumor-induced hypercalcemia were treated with a single infusion of APD. The mean age of the patients was 62 years (range 34–84 years). They suffered from the following tumors: 25 breast cancers, 20 squamous cell cancers, 5 myelomas, 4 prostate cancers, 4 undifferentiated lung cancers, and 10 of various histologies. After rehydration for 2 days, all the patients received a single infusion of APD (supplied by CIBA-GEIGY) with four different doses: 32 patients received 30 or 45 mg (low dose), and 36 patients received 60 or 90 mg (high dose), given over 24 h in 1 liter 0.9% saline solution, and with no other treatment for hypercalcemia.

Figure 2 shows the decrease of plasma calcium in the 68 patients over 2 weeks after the single infusion of APD. On average, plasma calcium decreased from 3.50 (±0.7) to 2.68 (±0.09) after 4 days, to 2.47 (±0.04) after 6 days, to 2.43 (±0.04) after 9 days, and to 2.48 (±0.04) after 14 days (mean ± SEM) (all in mmol/liter, and all $P < 0.001$ compared with the initial values). A dose response effect could

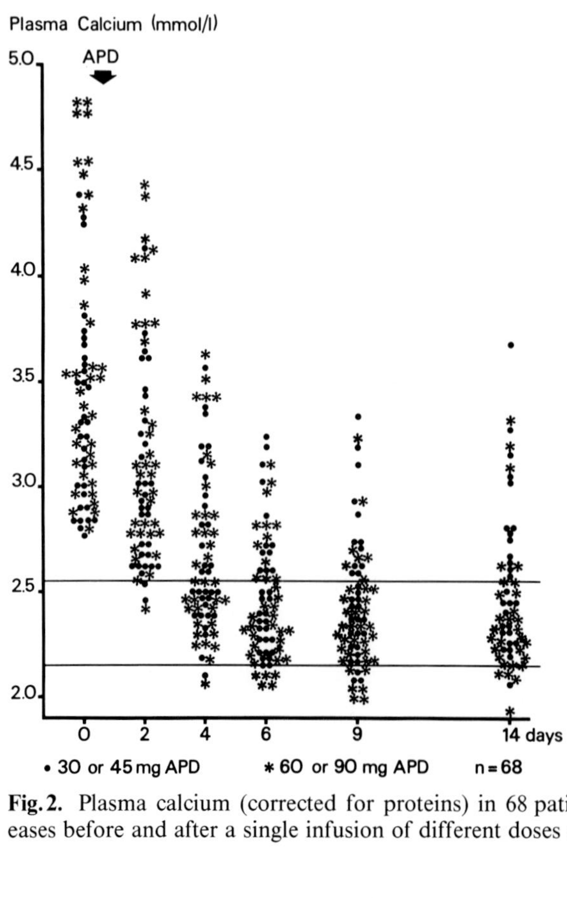

Fig. 2. Plasma calcium (corrected for proteins) in 68 patients with various malignant diseases before and after a single infusion of different doses of APD on day 0

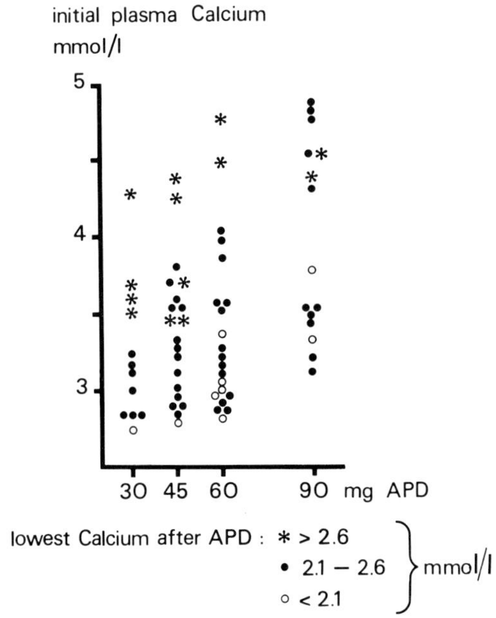

Fig. 3. Influence of the initial plasma calcium level (corrected) and of the dose of APD on the short-term result of the treatment. Low doses are insufficient in severe hypercalcemia, and high doses cause transient hypocalcemia in mild cases

be observed with more patients of the low-dose group reaching only the upper normal range or showing a trend to relapse after 9 days. Thirteen patients did not normalize their plasma calcium, nine of which belong to the low-dose group. Conversely, nine patients had a slight and asymptomatic hypocalcemia, of which seven belong to the high-dose group. The initial plasma calcium level predetermined the effect of a given dose, severe hypercalcemia needing higher doses for normalization than mild hypercalcemia (Fig. 3).

Figure 4 shows the 9-month follow-up of four groups of ten patients each, treated with different doses of APD, with respect to mortality and recurrence of hypercalcemia. Although the number of patients who died was almost identical at any time in the four groups, relapses of hypercalcemia occurred earlier and more frequently in the groups treated with the low dose of APD (30 or 45 mg). The biological parameters of excessive bone resorption fell dramatically after APD: after 6 days, urinary calcium was decreased by 80% and urinary hydroxyproline by 35%.

This study not only showed the effectiveness of the single-infusion regimen, but also demonstrated differences in short- and long-term effect due to the doses. Such differences were not evident for most authors, who administered bisphosphonates for at least 1 week, possibly using higher doses than necessary. By a shortening of the treatment to 3 days (Body et al. 1987) or to 1 day as in this study, the dose response could be demonstrated.

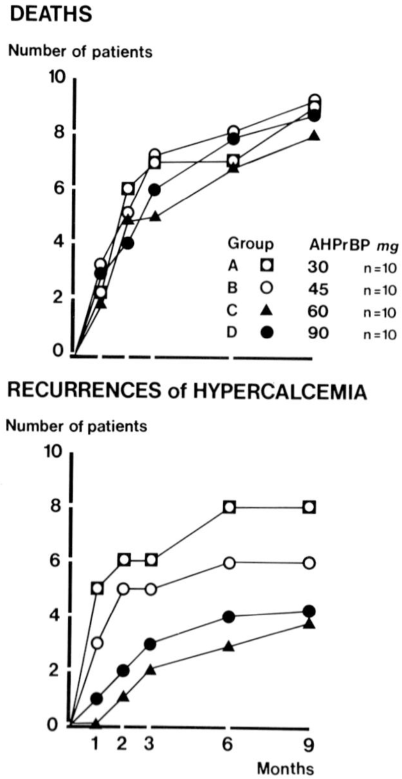

Fig. 4. Mortality and recurrence rate of hypercalcemia in four groups of ten patients with various cancer diseases, treated with different doses of APD (at time 0 and in the case of recurrence), and followed for 9 months. (Reprinted with permission of the *Journal of Clinical Oncology*)

Supportive Treatment for Bone Metastases in Breast Cancer (Phase II Trial)

Introduction

Metastases from breast cancer can cause bone pain, fractures, and hypercalcemia. The incidence of bone metastases depends to a large extent on the stage of the tumor at the time of diagnosis and ranges between 25% and 75% in patients with stage III disease (Elte et al. 1986; Paterson 1987). Severe morbidity from breast cancer may be essentially caused by pains due to bone involvement. As general and local osteolysis is a serious complication of breast carcinoma, the possibility of using bisphosphonates as supportive therapy has been raised. Few pilot studies have demonstrated a protective effect of a long-term treatment with oral bisphosphonates (Cl_2MBP or APD) in patients with bone metastases due to breast or other cancer (Adami et al. 1985; Chantraine et al. 1984; Delmas et al. 1982; Elomaa et al. 1983; Van Holten-Verzandvoort et al. 1987). The use of bisphosphonate was associated with a reduction in the urinary excretion of calcium and hydroxyproline suggesting an inhibition of bone resorption (Delmas et al. 1984; Siris et al. 1983; Van Holten-Verzandvoort et al. 1987). Moreover, in a controlled study (Elomaa et al. 1983, 1985), patients receiving bisphosphonates experienced fewer episodes of hypercalcemia, developed fewer bone lesions, and used less analgesics than the control group. But controlled follow-up studies in cancer patients are complicated by the responses to successive and concomitant hormone treatment, chemotherapy, and ethical difficulties.

Method

On the basis of the impressive effectiveness of single infusion of APD in hypercalcemia of malignancy, 25 normocalcemic patients suffering from advanced breast cancer with painful osteolytic bone metastases received intermittent (1- to 3-month intervals) intravenous infusions of 60 mg APD as a supportive therapy, without changing the previous hormonochemotherapy. The presence of extensive bone metastases was confirmed by conventional radiography and by scintigraphy, performed initially and every 3 months thereafter, and evaluated blind by a radiologist. All patients were referred by the oncologist, and had progressive disease but not more than one type of previous chemotherapy or hormonotherapy. Biological and clinical parameters were evaluated every month: plasma calcium, phosphorus, creatinine and serum proteins, urinary calcium, creatinine and hydroxyproline in 2-h morning urine sample, with methods previously described (Thiébaud et al. 1986a).

Pain score was examined by a specialist, according to a questionnaire with a usual pain scale, and drug changes for pain treatment were recorded as well.

APD was given at the dose of 60 mg at monthly intervals for 3 months, and thereafter every trimester, as a 24-h continuous infusion using a portable infusor (Travenol R, provided by Travenol Laboratories, Inc. Deerfield, Illinois, USA). The syringe pump contains exactly 60 ml (=60 mg APD), which is delivered slowly and continuously over 24 h through a catheter fixed in the arm, allowing the patient to live normally at home.

Results

Due to early death or to progression of the neoplastic disease necessitating a change in chemotherapy, only 13/25 patients with a mean age of 59 years (range 37–85 years) had a follow-up long enough to be eligibile for the study after 2 years. The patients are described in Table 3. They had a minimum of four courses APD and a mean follow-up of 11 months (range 6–18 months). Plasma calcium decreased from 2.51 ($\pm$0.05) mmol/liter to 2.40 ($\pm$0.04) ($P<0.01$) 6 months after APD treatment. No hypercalcemia occurred. Plasma creatinine and phosphate remained unchanged; urinary hydroxyproline and calcium are shown in Fig. 5. The marked fall with normalization of urinary calcium excretion (65% after 1 month and 42% after 6 months) and of urinary hydroxyproline excretion (about 35% over 6 months) (both with $P<0.001$) suggest a major reduction in the excessive bone resorption rate, confirming the efficacy of a single infusion of APD, as previously reported in hypercalcemia of malignancy.

Clinical improvement was assessed by the decrease in bone pain (Table 3), which was noted in 9/13 patients, with a mean remission of bone pain during

Table 3. Thirteen patients with breast cancer

Patient No.	Age (years)	Follow-up (months)	Follow-up[a]	Remission of pain	Radiological score[b]	Anticancer treatment
1	56	12	Progressive disease	–	1+2	Aminoglutethimide
2	64	6	Progressive disease	–	1+2	Aminoglutethimide
3	49	6	Progressive disease	–	1+2	Progestative
4	45	6	Progressive disease	–	1+2	4-Epiadriamycin
5	70	6	Progressive disease	+(3)	2	Progestative
6	68	9	No change	+(7)	2	Tamoxifen
7	47	14	Partial remission (10)	+(8)	1+3	Ovariectomy
8	56	18	Partial remission (12)	+(15)	3	Tamoxifen
9	54	7	Partial remission (5)	+(5)	3	Progestative
10	73	10	Progressive disease	+(10)	3	Tamoxifen
11	63	12	Progressive disease	+(9)	3	CMF[c]
12	85	6	No change	+(6)	1+3	Radiotherapy
13	37	14	Partial remission (11)	+(11)	3	Ovariectomy

[a] Partial remission (months).
[b] *1*, progressive lysis; *2*, normal sclerosis of metastases; *3*, intense sclerosis of metastases.
[c] Cyclophosphamide methotrexate fluorouracil.

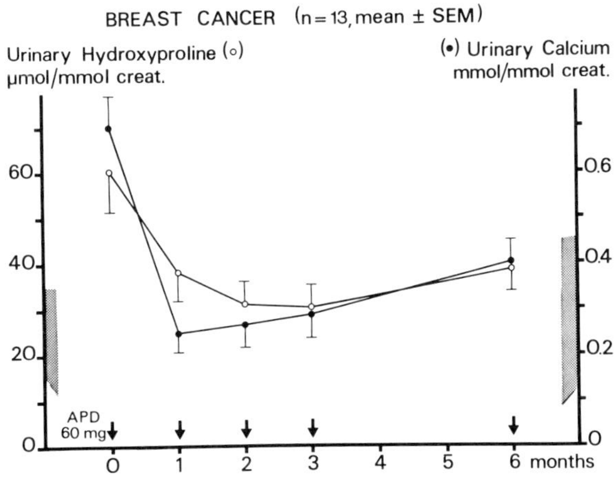

Fig. 5. Urinary hydroxyproline and calcium excretion in 13 patients with breast carcinoma and bone metastases during treatment with repeated infusions of 60 mg APD

9 months. The performance status improved similarly in these 9/13 patients, reading a mean score of 70%–80% according to the Karnofsky scale. Disease status (Table 3) was assessed on the basis of all clinical and paraclinical examinations and showed a progressive disease in 7/13 patients (new liver metastases in three and skin, brain, or pleural involvement in two patients); a partial remission in 4/13 patients (mean duration 9 months); and no change in 2/13 patients. Various concomitant anticancer treatments are indicated in Table 3 and no change occurred during the period of evaluation. The remission of pain in as many as 9/13 patients is noticeable because it occurred in 3 patients with progressive disease, in 2 patients with no change, and in 4 patients concomitantly with partial remission, suggesting a benefit from APD treatment, especially in the former. The important sclerosis of metastases in more than half of the patients also suggests a positive calcium balance due to decrease in local and general resorption.

No side effects could be observed except in two cases with transient moderate phlebitis at the beginning of the study due to the use of too short catheters. No fever or hematological side effects occurred.

Although this study does not prove that APD can prevent the progression of bone metastases, it evokes some beneficial effect on bone pain and densification of bone metastases, and it shows a marked decrease in the biological parameters of bone resorption. Moreover, the intravenous use of bisphosphonate appeared to be safe, allowing treatment of outpatients and optimizing bioavailability and compliance.

Conclusion

Due to its strong and sustained inhibitory effect on bone resorption, APD is a safe, well-tolerated, and highly efficient drug against malignant hypercalcemia when given intravenously. It has been used in over 350 patients. It normalized plasma calcium in almost all cases when appropriate doses were given, except in some cases of end-stage cancer disease. Its effect is dose dependent. Extremely severe hypercalcemia requires higher doses and more time for normalization, the slope of the drop of plasma calcium being almost constant. Its effect is prolonged, even when given in a single infusion. When hypercalcemia reoccurs, on average after 3 weeks, sometimes only, after several months, it can be retreated. It occurs less frequently after treatment with relatively high doses. Preliminary results in normocalcemic patients with bone metastases of breast cancer show a protective effect on bone, also demonstrated by Cleton et al. in this symposium. Outpatients were treated with repeated 24-h infusions, using a portable Travenol pump, fixed on the arm. Therefore, intravenous treatment with APD as a single or repeated infusion has been shown to be a highly efficient treatment of tumor-induced osteolysis in hospitalized patients and in ambulatory care.

Summary

Bisphosphonates, associated with rehydration, became the treatment of choice of malignant hypercalcemia when it became apparent that these compounds normalized plasma calcium in most cases within a few days and with almost no side effects, and that their effect was prolonged. Dichloromethylene bisphosphonate and aminobisphosphonate, especially APD, were shown to inhibit bone resorption with no noticeable inhibition of bone formation, and were highly effective in the long-term treatment of Paget's disease. APD was used in almost 300 patients with malignant hypercalcemia published in the literature and has been used in the medical clinic at Lausanne for several years. When given to 14 patients with malignant hypercalcemia at the dose of 25 mg/day until plasma calcium became normal for two consecutive days, APD had to be given for 4–11 days, severe hypercalcemia needing longer treatment than mild hypercalcemia (Adami et al. 1982). When given for a fixed period of 6 days, again plasma calcium normalized in all patients, whether APD was given i.v. (30 mg/day, ten patients) or orally (1200 mg/day, ten patients) (Adami et al. 1985). Further shortening of the treatment to one single infusion given over 24 h did not decrease the efficacy, as long as high enough doses were given (Blomqvist 1986). For severe hypercalcemia of above 3.5 mmol/liter 60–90 mg had to be given, while 30–45 mg was sufficient in milder cases (Body 1984). Otherwise, mild, transient, and asymptomatic hypocalcemia could occur. Normalization of plasma calcium went along with clinical improvement, sometimes even with correction of coma. Renal function was improved, even when the initial plasma creatinine levels were up to twice normal. Hypercalcemia could reoccur, but the duration of the effect of APD (1 week to several months) depended among other things on the dose administered. The decrease in plasma calcium was accompanied by a decrease in urinary calcium and hydroxyproline, both showing inhibition of bone resorption. In the case of recurrency, the treatment could be repeated with almost unaltered efficacy, except in end-stage cancer disease.

When given to 13 normocalcemic patients with bone metastases from breast cancer, hydroxyproline and urinary calcium again decreased. Bone pains and radiologic signs of metastatic bone resorption also showed significant improvement, although these latter effects could also be explained by the antitumoral treatment, in this uncontrolled open trial. But the biochemical follow-up over 6 months showed that the intravenous infusion of 60 mg APD with a portable Travenol pump, once every 1–3 months, in ambulatory outpatients exerted a noticeable inhibitory effect on bone resorption in these patients.

References

Adami S, Frijlink WB, Bijvoet OLM, O'Riordan JLH, Clemens TL, Papapoulos SE (1982) Regulation of calcium absorption by 1,25 dihydroxy-vitamin D – studies of the effects of a bisphosponate treatment. Calcif Tissue Int 34: 317–320

Adami S, Salvagno G, Guarrera G, Bianchi G, Dorizzi R, Rosini S, Mobilio G, Lo Cascio V (1985) Dichloromethylene-diphosphonate in patients with prostatic carcinoma metastatic to the skeleton. J Urol 134: 1152–1154

Blomqvist CP (1986) Malignant hypercalcemia. A hospital survey. Acta Med Scand 220: 455–463

Body JJ (1984) Cancer hypercalcemia: recent advances in understanding and treatment. Eur J Cancer Clin Oncol 20 (no 7): 865–869

Body JJ, Borkowski A, Cleeren A, Bijvoet OLM (1986) Treatment of malignancy-associated hypercalcemia with intravenous aminohydroxypropylidene diphosphonate. J Clin Oncol 4 (no 8): 1177–1183

Body JJ, Pot M, Borkowski M, Sculier JP, Klastersky J (1987) Dose-response study of aminohydroxypropylidene bisphosphonate in tumor-associated hypercalcemia. Am J Med 82: 957–963

Cantwell BMJ, Harris AL (1987) Effect of single high dose infusions of aminohydroxypropylidene diphosphonate on hypercalcaemia caused by cancer. Br Med J 294: 467–469

Chantraine A, Jung A, Van Quwenaller C, Donath A (1984) Le dichlorométhylène-diphosphonate dans le traitement des métastases osseuses lytiques. Presse Med 13 (no 8): 479–482

Coleman RE, Rubens RD (1987) APD for hypercalcaemia of breast cancer. Br J Cancer

Delmas PD, Charhon S, Chapuy MC, Vignon E, Briancon D, Edouard C, Meunier PJ (1982) Long-term effects of dichloromethylene diphosphonate (Cl_2MDP) on skeletal lesions in multiple myeloma. Metab Bone Dis Rel Res 4: 163–168

Elomaa I, Blomqvist C, Gröhn P, Porkka L, Kairento AL, Selander K, Lamberg-Allardt C, Holmström T (1983) Long-term controlled trial with diphosphonate in patients with osteolytic bone metastases. Lancet 1: 146–149

Elomaa I, Blomqvist C, Porkka L, Holmström T, Taube T, Lamberg-Allardt C, Borgström GH (1985) Diphosphonates for osteolytic metastases. Lancet 1: 1155–1156

Elte JWF, Bijvoet OLM, Cleton FJ, Van Oosterom AT, Sleeboom HP (1986) Osteolytic bone metastases in breast carcinoma pathogenesis, morbidity and bisphosphonate treatment. Eur J Cancer Clin Oncol 22 (no 4): 493–500

Fisken RA, Heath DA, Bold AM (1980) Hypercalcaemia – a hospital survey. Q J Med 196: 405–418

Harinck HIJ, Bijvoet OLM, Blanksma HJ, Dahlinghaus-Nienhuys PJ (1987a) Efficacious management with aminobisphosphonate (APD) in Paget's disease of bone. Clin Orthop Rel Res 217: 79–98

Harinck HIJ, Bijvoet OLM, Plantingh JST, Body JJ, Elte JWF, Sleeboom HP, Wildiers H, Neijt HP (1987b) Role of bone and kidney in tumor-induced hypercalcemia and its treatment with bisphosphonate and sodium chloride. Am J Med 82: 1133–1142

Jodrell DI, Iveson TJ, Smith IE (1987) Symptomatic hypocalcemia after treatment with high-dose aminohydroxypropylidene diphosponate. The Lancet 1: 622

Mundy GR (1985) Pathogenesis of hypercalcaemia of malignancy. Clin Endocrinol (Oxf) 23: 705–714

Mundy GR, Ibbotson KJ, D'Souza SM et al (1984) The hypercalcemia of cancer. Clinical implications and pathogenic mechanisms. N Engl J Med: 1718-1727

Papapoulos SE, Harinck HIJ, Bijvoet OLM, Gleed JH, Franer LJ, O'Riordan JLH (1986) Effects of decreasing serum calcium on circulating parathyroid hormone and vitamin D metabolites in normocalcaemic and hypercalcaemic patients treated with APD. Bone Mineral 1: 69-78

Paterson AHG (1987) Bone metastases in breast cancer, prostate cancer and myeloma. Bone 8 [Suppl 1]: S17-S22

Portmann L, Häfliger JM, Bill G, Burckhardt P (1983) Un traitement simple de l'hypercalcémie tumorale: l'amino-hydroxypropylidène bisphosphonate (APD) i.v. Schweiz Med Wochenschr 113: 1960-1963

Ralston SH, Gardner MD, Dryburgh FJ, Jenkins AS, Cowan RA, Boyle I (1985) Comparison of aminohydroxypropylidene diphosphonate, mithramycin and corticosteroids/calcitonin in treatment of cancer-associated hypercalcemia. Lancet 2: 907-910

Ralston SH, Alzaid AA, Gardner MD, Boyle IT (1986) Treatment of cancer associated hypercalcaemia with combined aminohydroxypropylidene diphosponate and calcitonin. Br Med J 292: 1549-1550

Siris ES, Hyman GA, Canfield RE (1983) Effects of dichloromethylene diphosphonate in women with breast carcinoma metastatic to the skeleton. Am J Med 74: 401-406

Sleebom HP, Bijvoet OLM, Van Oosterom AT et al (1983) Comparison of intravenous (3-amino-1-hydroxypropylidene)-1-bisphosphonate and volume repletion in tumour-induced hypercalcemia. Lancet ii 1: 239-243

Sleebom HP, Bijvoet OLM (1985) Treatment of tumour-induced hypercalcaemia. In: Garattini S (ed) Bone resorption, metastasis, and diphosphonates. Raven, New York, pp 59-78

Stevens MJ (1987) Efficacy of aminohydroxypropylidene diphosponate in the treatment of malignancy-associated hypercalcaemia. Med J Aust 146: 261-263

Thiébaud D, Jaeger P Jacquet AF, Burckhardt P (1986a) A single-day treatment of tumor-induced hypercalcemia by intravenous amino-hydroxypropylidene bisphosphonate. J Bone Min Res 1 (no 6): 555-562

Thiébaud D, Portmann L, Jaeger P, Jacquet AF, Burckhardt P (1986b) Oral versus intravenous AHPrBP (APD) in the treatment of hypercalcemia of malignancy. Bone 7: 247-253

Thiébaud D, Jaeger P, Burckhardt P (1987) Paget's disease of bone treated in five days with AHPrBP (APD) per os. J Bone Min Res 2 (no 1): 45-52

Thiébaud D, Jaeger P, Jacquet AF, Burckhardt P (1988) Dose response in the treatment of malignant hypercalcemia by a single infusion of the bisphosphonate AHPrBP (APD). J Clin Oncol 6: 762-768

Van Breukelen FJM, Bijvoet OLM, Van Oosterom AT (1979) Inhibition of osteolytic bone lesions by (3-amino-1-hydroxypropyledene)-1, 1-bisphosphonate (APD). Lancet 1: 803-805

Van Holten-Verzandvoort A, Harinck HIJ, Hermans J, Cleton FJ, Bijvoet OLM (1987) Supportive bisphosphonate treatment reduces morbidity from bone lesions in breast cancer. (abstract 390) 9th annual scientific meeting ASBMR, Indianapolis, June 1987

Yates AJP, Murray RML, Jerums GJ, Martin TJ (1987) A comparison of single and multiple intravenous infusions of APD (3-amino-1-hydroxypropylidene-1, 1-bisphosphonate) in the treatment of hypercalcemia of malignancy. Treatment of hypercalcemia with APD. Submitted to Aust N Z J Med 17: 387-391

Clodronate Therapy of Metastatic Bone Disease in Patients with Prostatic Carcinoma

S. Adami and M. Mian

Istituto di Semeiotica e Nefrologia Medica, University of Verona, Verona and
Ist. Formacologia University of Pisa, Pisa, Italy

Introduction

More than 80% of patients with prostatic cancer have skeletal metastasis (Galasko 1981; Abrams et al. 1980). Although hormonal treatment can induce remission of some length, the final outcome is frequently progressive skeletal disease, despite orchiectomy and/or continuous hormone therapy. At this stage, the efficacy of cytotoxic drugs is limited (Posner et al. 1977) and radiation therapy is used only in persons with epidural spinal cord compression. High-dose corticosteroids can produce a short-lasting reduction in symptoms (Yagoda 1983), which should be ascribed to a diminution of the inflammatory reaction around the metastatic lesion.

In 1985 (Adami et al. 1985) we showed in an uncontrolled study that dichloromethylene bisphosphonate or clodronate, a powerful inhibitor of bone resorption, may represent an important form of supporting treatment in patients with bone metastasis owing to prostatic carcinoma, providing sustained relief of pain: four patients who had been bedridden became ambulatory and reversal of paralysis was also noted in one of the patients. Similar results in small groups of patients treated with bisphosphonates have been reported by others (Percival et al. 1985; Schnur 1984; Urwin et al. 1985). Here we summarize our further experience on this issue.

Open Multicenter Trial

In the past 3 years we have collected data referring to a group of patients with prostatic tumors metastatic to the skeleton, treated with 300 mg clodronate i.v. for 10 days by several urologists or oncologists. The criteria for patient selection were: (a) radiographic evidence of bone metastasis; (b) orchiectomy performed at least 8 months before the treatment course; (c) extramustine therapy, but the patients had to enter the study at a time when the disease was progressive despite continuous treatment. Along with vials of clodronate, the physicians were provided with a questionnaire in which the main anamnestic, biochemical, and subjective findings had to be reported. Out of 92 patients, 80 experienced a dramatic improvement of pain; in the remaining 12, the physicians had some doubt about the bone origin of pain. Sixty patients were retreated as soon as pain recurred without any apparent

Recent Results in Cancer Research, Vol. 116

loss of efficacy. Most important of all, for an overall follow-up of 42 patient-years, hematological toxicity was never reported. Although the results with intravenous clodronate are, in the experience of several investigators, dramatically beneficial, a controlled study is still warranted since the efficacy of treatment relies mainly on changes in bone pain, which are difficult to evaluate. Furthermore the optimal duration and method of administration in order to prevent the relapse of pain still has to be defined.

Controlled Studies

Fifty-six patients with bone metastasis owing to prostatic carcinoma were randomly allocated to four single-blind controlled therapeutic protocols (see below). Eighteen patients underwent orchiectomy at least 8 months before entering the study. Sixteen patients were on extramustine therapy but they entered the study at a time when the disease was clearly progressive despite continuing therapy. The intensity of bone pain was assessed by the daily consumption of analgesic drugs (ketoprofen) and a visual analogue scale (20-cm line) graded from 0 (no pain) to 20 (extremely severe pain). Routine biochemical measurements on serum specimens were determined before treatment and at least once a month thereafter.

Placebo Versus Intravenous Clodronate

Thirteen patients were randomly allocated to either placebo (500 ml saline solution; $n=6$) or 300 mg clodronate dissolved in 500 ml saline solution infused daily intravenously over a period of 2 h for 2 weeks ($n=7$). The difference as regards both pain and analgesic consumption (Fig. 1) between the placebo and the clodronate group was so striking that we did not extend this trial for ethical reasons. Thus all patients on placebo were given clodronate intravenously and they are further described in the "maintenance protocol."

Oral Versus Intramuscular Clodronate

Twelve patients were given 100 mg clodronate/day intramuscularly for 2 weeks. The injections were rather painful but local induration was never observed. A significant fall in analgesic consumption was observed but not in pain as measured by the visual analogue scale (Fig. 2). In 11 patients 1200 mg clodronate per os, per day for 2 weeks in fasting conditions (2–3 h before breakfast) was completely ineffective (Fig. 2).

Maintenance Therapy

In the 13 patients given clodronate intravenously for 2 weeks pain relapsed fairly soon (Fig. 3). These results were compared with those observed in 18 patients given a maintenance therapy with 1200 mg clodronate/day for at least 6 weeks

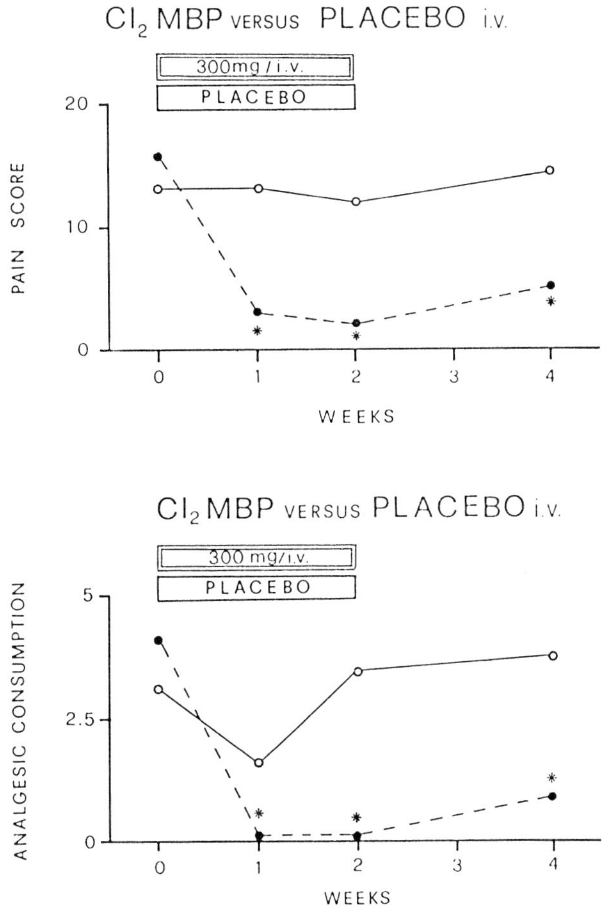

Fig. 1. Mean changes in pain score *(upper)* and analgesic consumption *(lower)* in six placebo-treated patients *(continuous line)* and in seven patients treated with intravenous clodronate *(interrupted line)*. * $P<0.01$ (paired t-test)

after a 2-week intravenous treatment course. This oral dose of clodronate, which was ineffective when given in the first place, seems to prevent the relapse of pain (Fig. 3).

Concluding Remarks

Pain due to metastatic bone disease often represents a major problem in the conservative treatment of patients with prostatic carcinoma. We believe that clodronate, which is now marketed in several countries, may represent the most effective supporting treatment in this condition. The intravenous route of administration (300 mg/day for at least 10 days) is required in order to obtain a rapid remission of pain, but oral administration (1200 or more mg/day) may be effective as a maintenance treatment.

In our experience clodronate therapy has never been associated with relevant hematological abnormalities; during treatment, a fall in urinary hydroxyproline

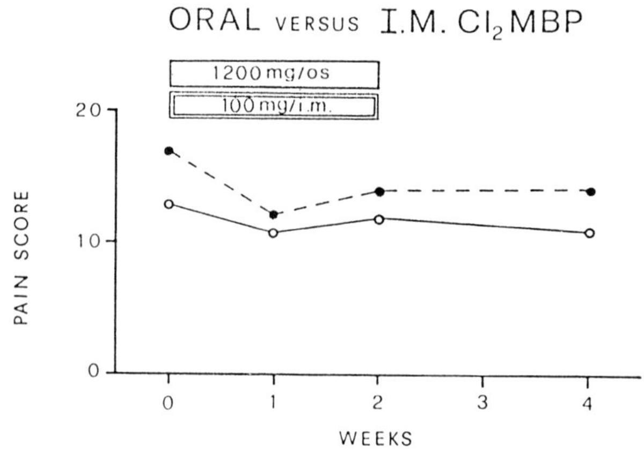

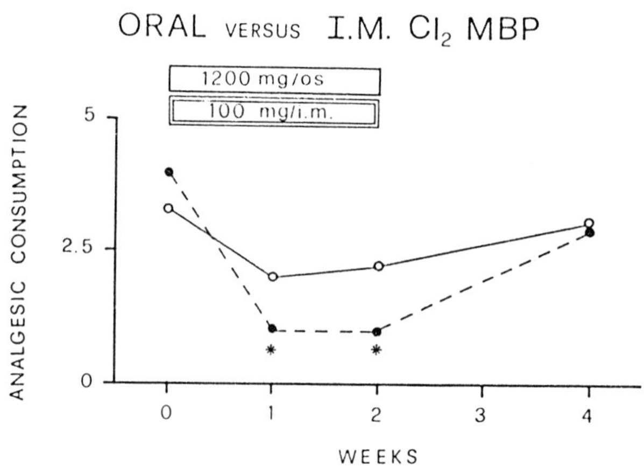

Fig. 2. Mean changes in pain score *(upper)* and analgesic consumption *(lower)* in patients treated with oral clodronate *(continuous line)* or with intramuscular clodronate *(interrupted line).*
* $P < 0.05$ (paired *t*-test)

and urinary calcium is observed, as expected; however, we did not notice any clear relationship between these biochemical changes and subjective symptoms. The results so far reported fully justify a prophylactic trial for the prevention of bone metastasis in patients with prostatic cancer.

Summary

Metastatic bone disease represents the most disabling complication in patients with prostatic carcinoma. In an open multicenter trial 80 out of 92 patients with bone metastasis due to prostatic carcinoma experienced a dramatic improvement of bone pain after treatment with 300 mg clodronate infused intravenously daily for 10 days. Further to this, 56 patients were randomly allocated to four single-blind controlled therapeutic trials, assessing bone pain by daily consumption of

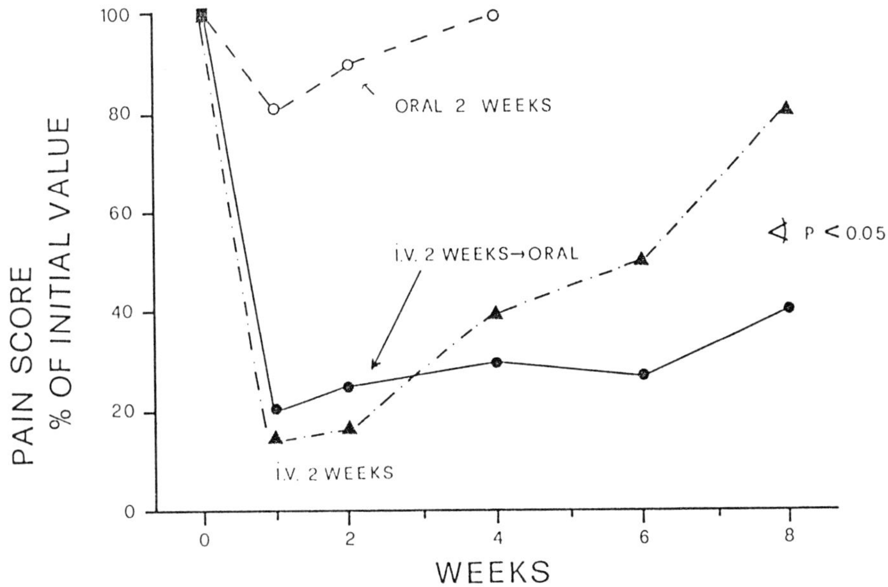

Fig. 3. Mean percentage changes in pain score in patients treated with clodronate. ○, 1200 mg/day orally for 2 weeks; ▲, 300 mg intravenously for 2 weeks; ●, 1200 mg orally after a 2-week treatment course with intravenous clodronate

analgesic drugs and by visual analogue scale. In the first protocol the effects of 2 weeks' treatment with intravenous infusion of either 300 mg clodronate dissolved in 500 ml saline (7 patients) or 500 ml saline (6 patients) were compared. The differences in both pain score and analgesic consumption were so striking that the trial was not extended for ethical reasons and all patients on placebo were given clodronate intravenously. Oral administration of 1200 mg clodronate for 2 weeks was completely ineffective in 11 patients. Intramuscular administration of 100 mg clodronate for 2 weeks induced in 12 patients a significant fall in analgesic consumption but not in the pain score. In most of the 13 patients given clodronate intravenously for 2 weeks bone pain relapsed fairly soon. However, in 18 patients a maintenance therapy with 1200 mg clodronate/day for at least 6 weeks after a 2-week intravenous treatment course did prevent the relapse of bone pain. In all patients given clodronate routine biochemical examination was carried out during and after treatment. For an overall follow-up of 42 patient-years hematologic toxicity was never observed. These results confirm that clodronate represents the most effective and convenient conservative treatment of patients with painful bone metastasis from prostatic carcinoma.

Acknowledgments. We wish to thank the several physicians who referred the patients to us and Istituto Gentili SpA for the supplies of clodronate.

References

Abrams HL, Spiro R, Goldstein N (1980) Metastasis in carcinoma: analysis of 1000 autopsied cases. Cancer 3: 74-85

Adami S, Salvagno G, Guarrera G, Bianchi G, Dorizzi R, Rosini S, Mobilio G, Lo Cascio V (1985) Dichloromethylene-diphosphonate in patients with prostatic carcinoma metastatic to the skeleton. J Urol 134: 1152-1154

Galasko C (1981) The anatomy and pathways of skeletal metastasis. In: Weiss L, Gilbert H (eds) Bone metastasis. G. K. Hall, Boston, pp 49-63

Percival RC, Watson ME, Williams JL, Kanis JA (1985) Carcinoma of the prostate: remission of paraparesis with inhibitor of bone resorption. Postgrad Med J 61: 551-553

Posner JB, Howieson J, Cvitkovic E (1977) "Disappearing" spinal cord compression: oncolytic effect of glucocorticoids (and other chemotherapeutic agents) on epidural metastasis. Ann Neurol 2: 409-413

Schnur W (1984) Etidronate for the relief of metastatic bone pain. J Urol 131: 404-407

Urwin GH, Percival RC, Harris S, Beneton MNC, William JL, Kanis JA (1985) Generalised increase in bone resorption in carcinoma of the prostate. Br J Urol 57: 721-723

Yagoda A (1983) Response in prostatic cancer: an enigma. Semin Urol 1: 311-323

Effect of Long-Term Bisphosphonate Treatment on Morbidity Due To Bone Metastases in Breast Cancer Patients

F.J. Cleton, A.T. van Holten-Verzantvoort, and O.L.M. Bijvoet

Department of Clinical Oncology, University Hospital Leiden, Building 1 K1-P, PO Box 9600, 2300 RC Leiden, The Netherlands

Breast cancer is the commonest type of cancer in European women. About half of the patients develop advanced disease following surgery. The majority of these patients suffer from osteolytic bone metastases at some time during the course of their disease (Elte et al. 1986). Hypercalcemia is a frequent complication in patients with extensive lesions in the skeleton. Osteolytic bone metastases cause severe morbidity and often incapacitate the patients.

Bisphosphonates are potent inhibitors of bone resorption and we therefore attempted to treat both hypercalcemia and osteolytic bone lesions with a bisphosphonate (Van Breukelen et al. 1979; van Holten-Verzantvoort et al. 1987). In these studies APD (3-amino-1-hydroxypropylidene-1,1-bisphosphonate), a compound developed in the Department of Endocrinology, University Hospital Leiden (Lemkes et al. 1978) and extensively used in the treatment of Paget's disease of the bone (Harinck et al. 1987b) was chosen. The qualitative effects of APD on calcium metabolism in tumor-induced hypercalcemia were examined in preliminary studies. Intravenous APD appears to be a simple and effective method for treating this condition (van Breukelen 1982; Mundy et al. 1983; Sleeboom et al. 1983).

The efficacy of APD as treatment for the hypercalcemia of malignancy was examined in a phase II multicenter study in 132 patients with a variety of malignant tumors, including 50 patients with breast cancer. APD was administered intravenously in a dose of 15 mg dissolved in 500 ml saline over 2 h. The infusions were repeated daily until 1 day after the normalization of the uncorrected serum calcium concentration. The serum calcium concentration was normalized within 5 days in more than 90% of the patients and in 48 of 50 patients with breast cancer. The median time to normalization was between 3 and 4 days. There were few side effects associated with intravenously administered APD, consisting of low-grade fever and a slight lymphopenia in a minority of patients.

It was expected that long-term administration of APD would be required to prevent and treat osteolytic lesions in patients with advanced breast cancer. For practical reasons an oral formulation of APD was developed. In a preliminary dose-finding study it was established that a daily dose of 300 mg APD was well tolerated by most patients. In this paper we summarize data from the interim analysis of a multicenter controlled trial of APD in patients with advanced breast cancer (Sleeboom et al. 1983).

Recent Results in Cancer Research, Vol. 116

Patients and Methods

Patients with hematogenous metastasis of breast cancer were randomized between treatment with APD or control. In the present report only patients with bone metastases will be considered. There were 70 patients in the APD-treated group and 61 patients as controls. The distribution of cases according to age, receptor status, distribution of bone metastases, previous hypercalcemia, and previous systemic treatment was similar in both groups. The inclusion and exclusion criteria are mentioned in Table 1.

APD was given as enteric-coated 150-mg tablets twice daily. A follow-up examination was carried out at 3 months. Bone scans and X-ray of the relevant lesions in the skeleton were performed every 6 months. The specific local or systemic tumor therapy was variable throughout the trial and left to the discretion of the patient's physician. At the time of the interim analysis the median follow-up was 13 months (range 1-36 months) for the APD group and 14 months (range 1-30 months) for the controls.

The APD treatment was intended to be continuous, without regard to the occurrence of events or increased skeletal morbidity. Hypercalcemia in both groups was to be treated with short courses of intravenous APD.

Follow-up and Analysis

There were 323 3-month evaluation intervals in the APD group and 297 such intervals in the controls. The following events were analyzed:

- Occurrence of hypercalcemia (serum calcium exceeding 2.75 mmol/liter)
- Bone pain, requiring radiotherapy or surgery
- Pathological or imminent fractures
- Number of changes in systemic treatment, because of progressive disease
- Number of local treatments for skeletal disease
- APD toxicity

Table 1. Patient inclusion and exclusion criteria

Inclusion	- Histologically confirmed breast cancer
	- Osteolytic metastases or/and advanced disease requiring systemic treatment
	- Advanced disease and progression under systemic treatment
Exclusion	- Gastrointestinal ulcers
	- Malabsorption
	- Pregnancy
	- Radiotherapy to the only evaluable lesion
	- Creatinine clearance less than 30 ml/min
	- Hypercalcemia
	- Other malignancy, except in situ cancer of the cervix and skin cancer other than melanoma
	- Expected poor compliance

The patients received an enquiry form concerning their quality of life at 3-month intervals. These have not been included in the interim analysis. Statistical analysis was made with the log-rank test and for comparison of some items with the Mann-Whitney test and the χ^2 test.

Results

All events related to skeletal morbidity, either occurring alone or as combined events, were considered as one complication within a single 3-month period. There were significantly more complications in the controls (67) than in the APD group (32). The total morbidity has been plotted as the cumulative sum of complications during successive observation intervals. The slopes thus obtained for both groups were approximately linear throughout the study. They represent the events per unit time and are a measure of morbidity (Fig. 1). With APD treatment morbidity more than halved. The occurrence of skeletal morbidity is shown in Table 2.

Hypercalcemia did not occur in the APD-treated group of patients, compared with 13 episodes in 8 patients in the control. Of the other events that were documented, all occurred significantly more frequently in the control group except for surgery, which was too infrequent for making meaningful conclusions.

Side Effects

In a pilot study using 600 mg APD daily, major toxicity was encountered, mainly consisting of nausea and vomiting. With half this dose nausea was limited to a minority of the patients causing a dropout rate of 8%. Many nongastrointestinal and nonskeletal effects were reported, which may have been compatible with breast cancer or the systemic treatment and are presently difficult to evaluate.

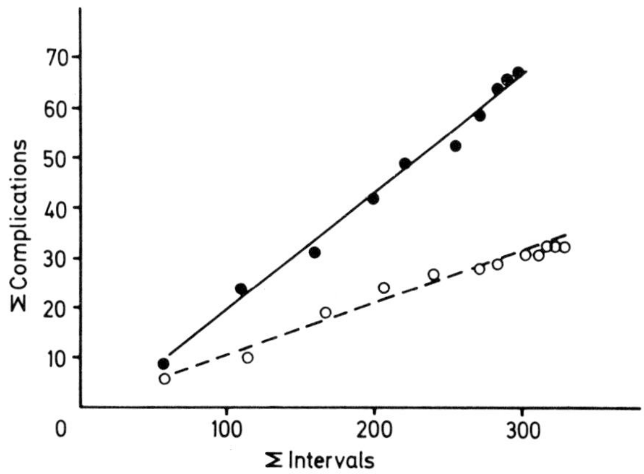

Fig. 1. Cumulative sum of complications per 3-month interval by cumulative sum of these intervals

Table 2. Occurrence of morbidity

Events	No. of events per patient				Total No. of events	*p* value
	0	1	2	⩾3		
Hypercalcemia						
APD	70[a]	0	0	0	0	<0.002
Controls	53	3	5	0	13	
Bone pain						
APD	60	9	1	0	11	<0.003
Controls	37	18	4	2	33	
Fractures and imminent fractures						
APD	67	3	0	0	3	<0.01
Controls	49	10	2	0	14	
Change of medication						
APD	47	20	2	1	27	<0.07
Controls	30	19	6	6	53	
Radiotherapy						
APD	60	9	1	0	11	<0.001
Controls	36	19	4	2	34	
Surgery						
APD	69	1	0	0	1	NS
Controls	58	2	1	0	4	
Complications[b]						
APD	42	25	2	1	32	<0.002
Controls	23	23	6	9	67	

NS, not significant.
[a] No. of patients.
[b] Isolated or combined events.

Discussion

Bisphosphonates are small molecules which bind to calcified bone matrix and inhibit osteoclastic bone resorption (Boonekamp et al. 1986; Boonekamp et al. 1987; Fleisch 1982; Lemkes et al. 1978). APD probably acts through inhibition of the attachment of osteoclasts to bone (Boonekamp et al. 1986; Boonekamp et al. 1987). Various types of bisphosphonates have been used in diseases with severe osteoclastic bone resorption (Fleisch 1982; Harinck et al. 1987a, b; Hoekman et al. 1985; Elomaa et al. 1983). The efficacy of oral and intravenous APD in Paget's disease and tumor hypercalcemia has been established by many investigators (Jung 1982). Several small controlled trials have been conducted in the treatment of metastatic bone disease (Delmas et al. 1984; Elomaa et al. 1983; Siris et al. 1983) with some suppression of morbidity.

In the present study of 131 patients, the interim analysis shows that APD treatment in addition to conventional systemic therapy more than halves the requirement for specific treatment of bone lesions. The treatment is simple and usually well tolerated. The incidence of pathological fractures and severe bone pain was reduced. Hypercalcemia was prevented in this group of patients. Morbidity caused by osteolytic metastases was not completely prevented and this poses questions about the adequacy of the chosen APD regimen relating to dose and duration of treatment. In this group of patients with a relatively short life expectancy we chose continuous treatment. In an adjuvant setting a decision should be made about the optimal duration of APD treatment, considering potential side effects in long-term survivors. The oral dose tolerated was equivalent (3 mg) to the low region of the dose-reponse relationship determined in a study on intravenous APD in Paget's disease (Harinck et al. 1987b). APD could be given in a considerably higher dose intravenously, but this is precluded for practical reasons.

The gastrointestinal side effects caused a withdrawal of 8% of patients from the study. Side effects are of great importance in supportive and adjuvant therapy. Efforts should therefore be made to develop more effective and less toxic bisphosphonates (Boonekamp et al. 1987). Such compounds should completely prevent complications from metastatic bone disease in patients with breast cancer.

Summary

The effect of long-term bisphosphonate (APD) treatment on the morbidity from bone metastases in breast cancer patients was studied in a controlled clinical trial. 131 patients were randomized between treatment with APD (300 mg/day orally) or control. Systemic treatment for breast cancer was left to the discretion of the physician. The distribution of cases according to age, receptor status and previous treatment was similar in both groups. Patients were examined at 3-month intervals, while bone scans and radiography of relevant lesions in the skeleton were performed every 6 months. After a median follow-up of 13 months, the morbidity in the treated group was significantly less than in the controls. This concerned the occurrence of hypercalcemia, bone pain and fractures, and the need for radiotherapy of osteolytic lesions. In this interim analysis, APD treatment more than halved the requirement for specific treatment of bone lesions. The treatment is simple and well tolerated at a relatively low dosage. A higher oral dose was precluded due to gastrointestinal toxicity. Because the effect of APD on skeletal morbidity was not complete, efforts should be made to develop more effective and less toxic bisphosphonates.

References

Boonekamp PM, van der Wee-Pals LJA, van Wijk-van Lennep MML, Thesingh CW, Bijvoet OLM (1986) Two modes of action of bisphosphonates on osteolytic resorption of mineralized bone matrix. Bone Mineral 1: 27–39

Boonekamp PM, van der Wee-Pals LJA, van Wijk-van Lennep MML, Bijvoet OLM (1987) Enhancement of the inhibitory action of APD on the transformation of osteoclast precursors into resorbing cells after dimethylation of the amino group. Bone Mineral 2: 29–42

Delmas PD, Charbon SA, Chapuy MC, Meunier PJ (1984) Place des diphosphonates dans le thérapeutique de l'ostéolyse et des hypercalcémiees malignes. Rev Rhum Mal Osteoartic 51: 663–666

Elomaa I, Blomquist C, Grôhn P (1983) Long-term controlled trial with diphosphonate in patients with ostelolytic bone metastases. Lancet 1: 146-149

Elomaa I, Blomquist C, Porrka L (1985) Diphosphonates for osteolytic metastases. Lancet 1: 1155-1156

Elte JWF, Bijvoet OLM, Cleton FJ, van Oosterom AT, Sleeboom WP (1986) Osteolytic bone metastasis in breast carcinoma: pathogenesis, morbidity and bisphosphonate treatment. Eur J Cancer Clin Oncol 22: 493-500

Fleisch H (1982) Bisphosphonates: mechanism of action and clinical applications. In: Peck WA (ed) Bone mineral research, vol I. Exerpta Medica, Amsterdam, pp 319-357

Harinck HIJ, Bijvoet OLM, Planting AST, Body JJ, Elte JWF, Sleeboom HP, Wildiers J, Neyt JP (1987a) Role of bone kidney in tumor-induced hypercalcemia and its treatment with bisphosphonate and sodium chloride. Am J Med 82: 1133-1142

Harinck HIJ, Bijvoet OLM, Blanksma HJ, Dahlinghaus-Nienhuys PJ (1987b) Efficacious management with APD in Paget's disease of bone. Clin Orthop Rel Res 217: 79-98

Hoekman K, Papapoulos SE, Bijvoet OLM (1985) Characteristics and bisphosphonate treatment of a patient with juvenile osteoporosis. J Clin Endocrinol Metab 61: 952-965

Jung A (1982) Comparison of two parenteral diphosphonates in hypercalcemia of malignancy. Am J Med 72: 221-226

Lemkes HPJJ, Reitsma PH, Frijlink WB (1978) A new bisphosphonate: dissociation between effects on cells and mineral in rats and a preliminary trial in Paget's disease. Adv Exp Med Biol 103: 459-569

Mundy GR, Wilkinson R, Heath DA (1983) Comparative study of available medical therapy for hypercalcemia of malignancy. Am J Med 74: 421-432

Siris ES, Hijman GA, Canfield ER (1983) Effects of dichloromethylene diphosphonate in women with breast carcinoma metastatic to the skeleton. Am J Med 74: 401-406

Sleeboom HP, Bijvoet OLM, van Oosterom AT, Eleed JH, O'Riddan JLM (1983) Efficacy of intravenous APD on serum calcium, magnesium and creatinine in tumour hypercalcaemia, compared with volume repletion. Lancet 2: 239-243

van Breukelen FJM, Bijvoet OLM, van Oosterom AT (1979) Inhibition of osteolytic bone lesions by APD. Lancet 1: 803-806

van Breukelen FJM, Bijvoet OLM, Frijlink WB, Sleeboom HP, Mulder H, van Oosterom AT (1982) Efficacy of APD in hypercalcaemia: observations on regulation of serum calcium. Calc Tiss Int 34: 321-327

van Holten-Verzantvoort ATh, Bijvoet OLM, Cleton FJ, Hermans J, Kroon HM, Harinck HIJ, Vermey P, Elte JWF, Neijt JP, Beex LVAM, Blijham G (1987) Reduced morbidity from skeletal metastases in breast cancer patients during long-term bisphosphonate (APD) treatment. Lancet 2: 983-985